ERCP
2nd edition
Color Illustration

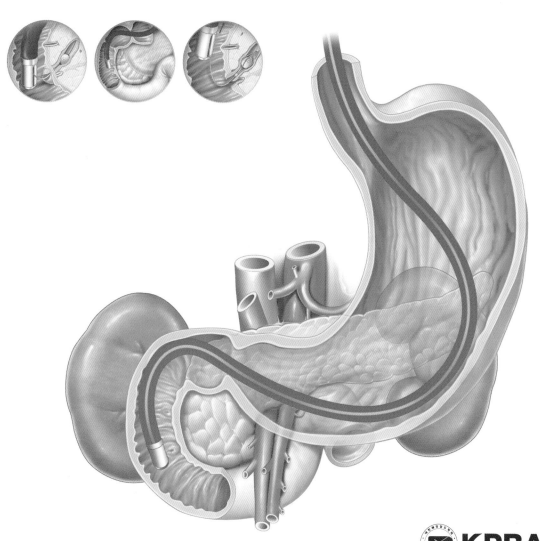

KPBA Korean
Pancreatobiliary
Association

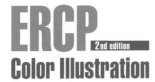

ERCP 2nd edition
Color Illustration

First edition published	April 27, 2009
Second edition printed	April 03, 2020
Second edition published	April 17, 2020

Written by	Korean Pancreatobiliary Association
Editor-in-chief	Kyo-Sang Yoo
Published by	Ju-yeon Jang
Planned by	Do-sung Kim
Edited by	Gyeong-hee An
Editing Design by	Eun-mi Joo
Cover Design by	Jae-wook Kim
Illustrations by	Ho-hyeon Lee
Produced by	Sang-hyeon Shin
Publishing House	Koonja Publishing Company
	Registration No. 4-139 (June 24, 1991)
	Paju Publishing Complex, 338, Hoedong-gil (474-1 Seopae-dong),
	Paju-si, Gyeonggi-do, South Korea (10881)
	Telephone : (031) 943-1888 Fax : (031) 955-9545
	Website : www.koonja.co.kr

ISBN   979-11-5955-562-6

ERCP Color Illustration

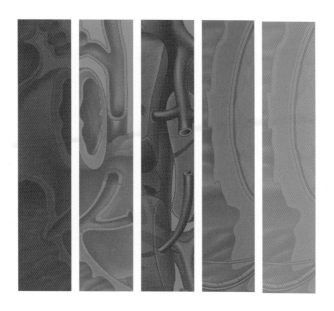

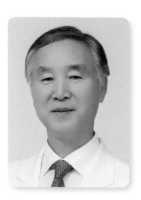

More than 10 years have passed since we published the first edition of ERCP illustration. Ever since it came out in 2009, this book has helped ERCP experts, fellows, residents, nurses, and medical students better understand the complex anatomical structures and physiological functions of the pancreatobiliary tract. It also aided in getting a solid grasp of the basic and complex techniques of pancreatobiliary endoscopy. This was made possible by depicting realistic endoscopic, ERCP and EUS photos, and also by adding schematic diagrams from a professional perspective.

During the past 10 years, new technologies and procedures such as interventional EUS have been introduce and developed in the field of pancreatobiliary intervention. Therefore, it was about time the Korean Pancreatobiliary Association released a second edition with better and more realistic pictures with the addition of latest endoscopic techniques and procedures. We believe that this second edition will provide clearer understanding in all aspects of pancreatobiliary system to the healthcare professionals.

I would like to express my sincere appreciation and congratulations to all the authors and the editor-in-chief who worked so hard to publish this wonderful book.

Ho Soon Choi, MD, PhD

President

Korean Pancreatobiliary Association

Foreword

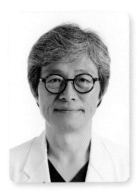

Congratulations on publishing the 2nd edition!

I believe that this book will significantly contribute to boosting up ERCP techniques to a higher level which the Korean Pancreatobiliary Association has continuously been pursuing. In addition, this book is expected to remarkably shorten the duration for ERCP beginners to become experts.

I am deeply grateful to all the authors and illustrators for their consistent efforts in making this book more up-to-date and simple.

Sang-Heum Park, MD

Chairman (2018)

Korean Pancreatobiliary Association

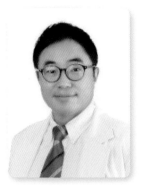

The pancreatobiliary tract has one of the most complicated structures and physiological functions in our body. Endoscopic procedure in this ductal system thus requires application of rather complicated techniques.

The first edition of this book was specifically written to overcome such difficulties by promoting better understanding and providing relevant medical information on pancreatobiliary lesions and pancreatobiliary endoscopy in the shortest time possible.

Many areas in the management of pancreatobiliary disorders have remarkably evolved, and new techniques including endoscopic ultrasound (EUS) guided interventions have emerged. In this second edition, you will not only become more familiar with the anatomy and diseases of the pancreatobiliary tract but also be able to understand various latest ERCP and EUS procedures with ease while looking at the detailed illustrations..

The authors painstakingly searched through the books, articles, and internet to find the most representative figures and images, all of which have been modified and redrawn one by one to make the best illustrations.

I would like to express my hearty thanks to all the authors for their exceptional contributions and to the artist who dedicated himself to elaborate computer graphics.

Seok Ho Dong, MD, PhD
Chairman (2019)
Korean Pancreatobiliary Association

Preface

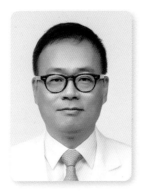

"A picture is worth a thousand words."

Performing endoscopic retrograde cholangiopancreatography (ERCP) needs comprehensive understanding of complex anatomical structures of pancreatobiliary system along with various techniques of ERCP. For this reason, illustrations can be much more informative than written material, especially for teaching and learning purposes.

The editors of this book are pleased to present the second edition of ERCP Color Illustration. The first edition was published in 2009 by wholehearted support of Korean Pancreatobiliary Association.

All the contents in this new edition have been updated by thoroughly reviewing every minute details from the previous edition with the intent to provide the readers with the most current and pertinent information on ERCP. As it had been with the previous edition, this updated edition continues to emphasize more detailed and realistic illustrations related to ERCP. We are confident that this book would prove to be highly useful not only to the endoscopists but also to other healthcare workers in getting relevant information instantly in ERCP suite.

In addition to updating the previous edition, new contents and chapters have been added. In Part 5 of this 2nd edition, new illustrations on several rescue procedures of ERCP, i.e. PTBD, PTCS, gallbladder drainage and recently popular procedure like EUS-guided bile duct drainage, have been included. Part 6 is a new chapter that illustrates ERCP accessories. Tables on accessories that are currently commercially available will help the readers better understand their specifications and characteristic features.

I am privileged to have worked with all enthusiastic editors who have put all their heart and soul into this book, and would truly like to express my deepest gratitude to them. I also would like to express my appreciation to the medical illustrator for their outstanding art work which significantly improved the figures, and also to the publisher for their great teamwork. We, all editors, hope that our readers will find this new edition to be highly informative resource in mastering ERCP.

Kyo-Sang Yoo, MD, PhD
Editor-in-Chief

Editors

Sang-Woo Cha, MD, PhD

Professor of Medicine
SoonChunHyang University Seoul Hospital, Seoul

Jae Hee Cho, MD, PhD

Professor of Medicine
Yonsei University Gangnam Severance Hospital, Seoul

Jong Jin Hyun, MD, PhD

Professor of Medicine
Korea University Ansan Hospital, Ansan

Dong Hee Koh, MD, PhD

Professor of Medicine
Hallym University Dongtan Sacred Heart Hospital, Hwaseong

Chang-il Kwon, MD, PhD

Professor of Medicine
CHA University CHA Bundang Medical Center, Seongnam

Sang Hyub Lee, MD, PhD

Professor of Medicine
Seoul National University Hospital, Seoul

Tae Hoon Lee, MD, PhD

Professor of Medicine
SoonChunHyang University Cheonan Hospital, Cheonan

Kyo-Sang Yoo, MD, PhD

Professor of Medicine
Hanyang University Guri Hospital, Guri

ERCP Color Illustration 2nd edition

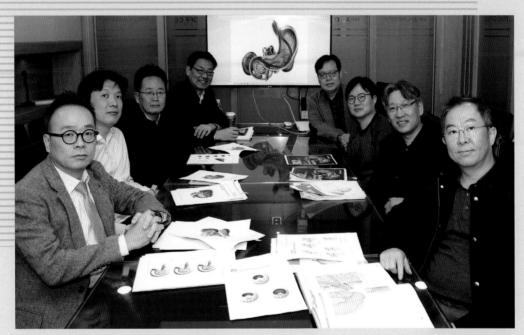

Editorial conference in March 2020

Contents

PART

I

Normal and Variant Anatomy of Pancreaticobiliary Tract

PART

II

Ampulla of Vater

PART

III Biliary Tract

PART

IV Pancreas

Contents

PART

V Techniques of ERCP

PART

VI ERCP Accessories

PART

I

Normal and Variant Anatomy of Pancreaticobiliary Tract

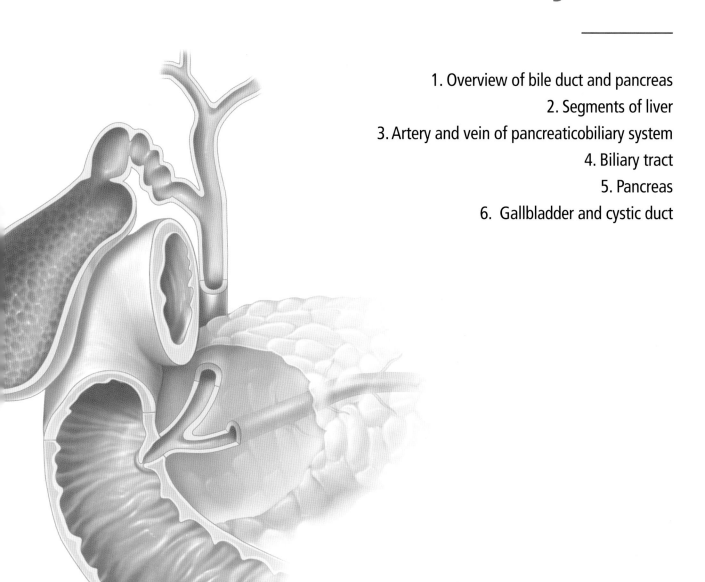

01 Overview of bile duct and pancreas

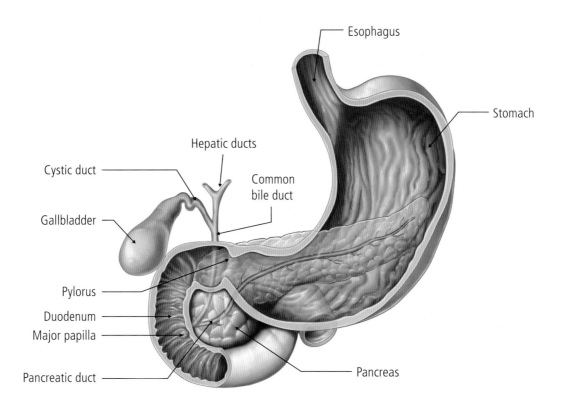

Esophagus

Stomach

Hepatic ducts

Cystic duct

Common bile duct

Gallbladder

Pylorus

Duodenum

Major papilla

Pancreatic duct

Pancreas

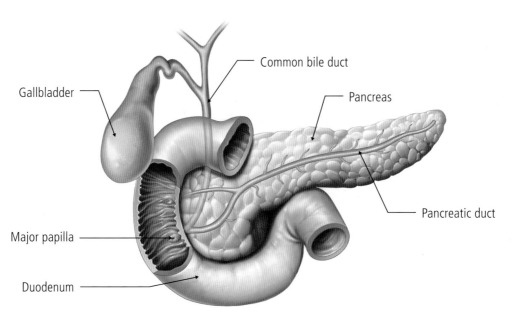

Common bile duct

Gallbladder

Pancreas

Major papilla

Pancreatic duct

Duodenum

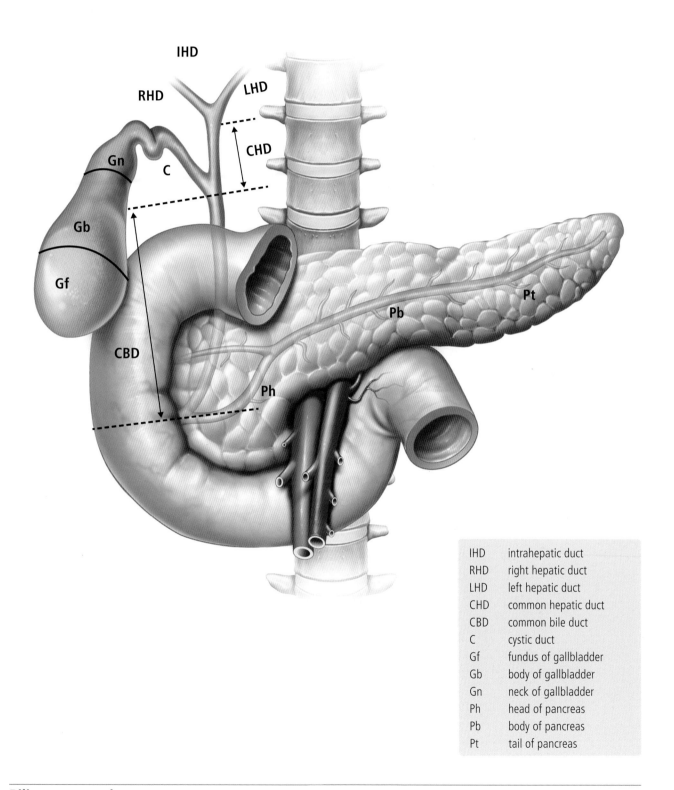

IHD	intrahepatic duct
RHD	right hepatic duct
LHD	left hepatic duct
CHD	common hepatic duct
CBD	common bile duct
C	cystic duct
Gf	fundus of gallbladder
Gb	body of gallbladder
Gn	neck of gallbladder
Ph	head of pancreas
Pb	body of pancreas
Pt	tail of pancreas

Biliary tract and pancreas

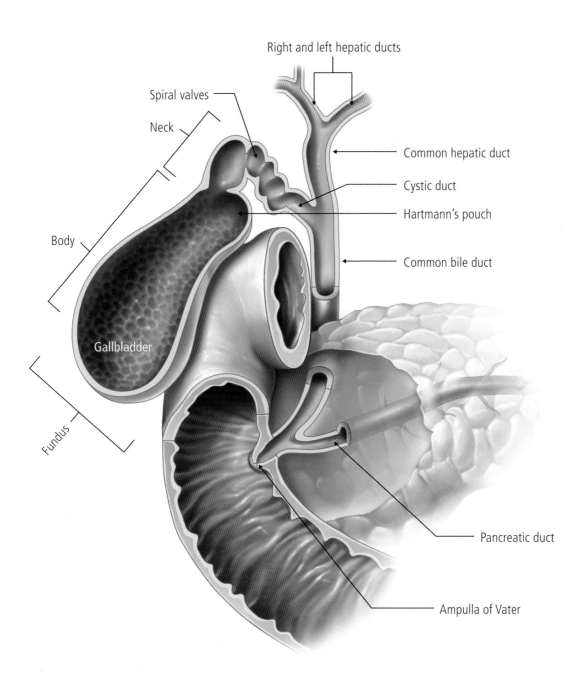

Right and left hepatic ducts

Spiral valves

Neck

Common hepatic duct

Cystic duct

Hartmann's pouch

Body

Common bile duct

Gallbladder

Fundus

Pancreatic duct

Ampulla of Vater

Gallbladder and bile duct

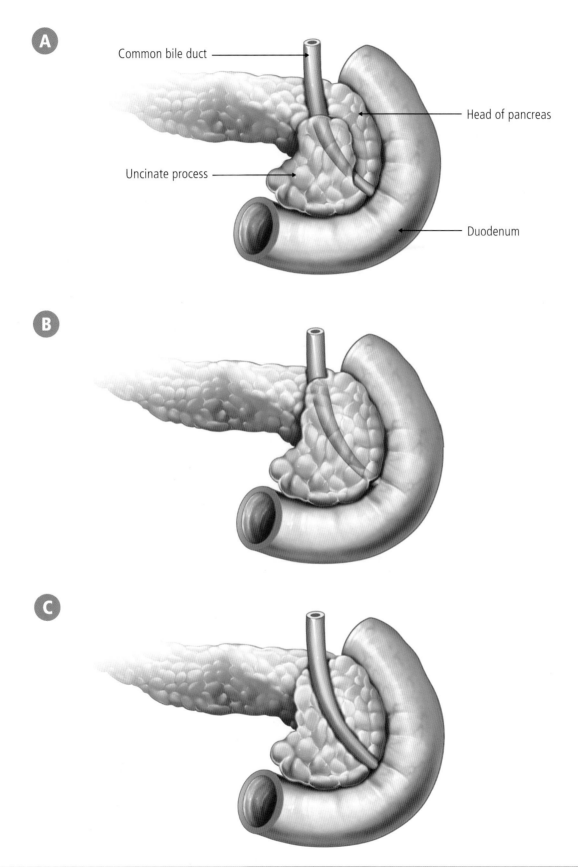

A

Common bile duct

Head of pancreas

Uncinate process

Duodenum

B

C

Variation of distal common bile duct, posterior view

02 / Segments of liver

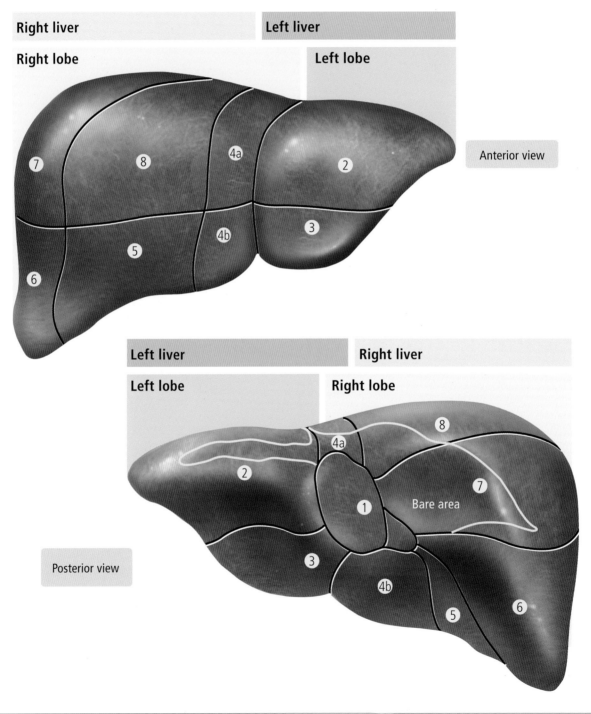

Right liver

Right lobe

Left liver

Left lobe

Anterior view

7 8 4a 2 3 4b 5 6

Left liver

Left lobe

Right liver

Right lobe

Posterior view

8 4a 2 7 1 Bare area 3 4b 5 6

Segments of liver

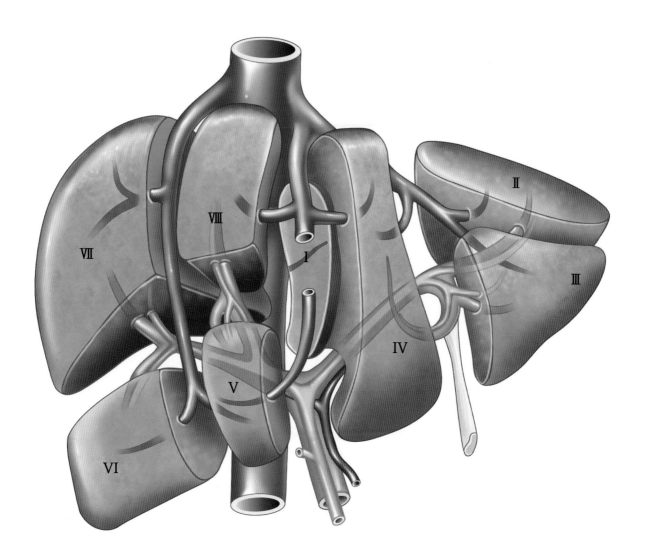

Functional division of liver segments according to Couinaud's nomenclature

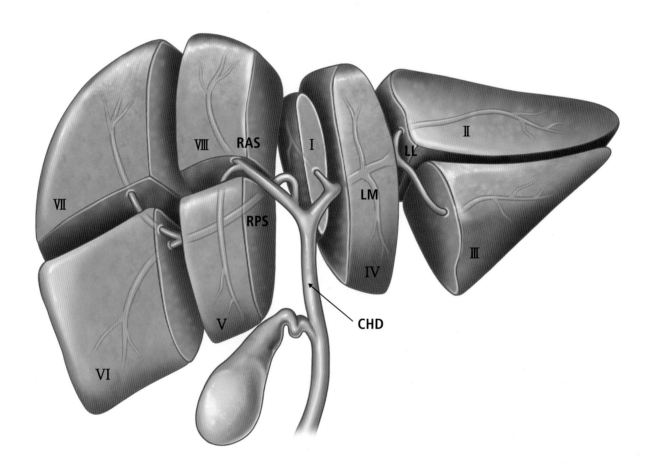

CHD	common hepatic duct
RPS	right posterior segmental duct
RAS	right anterior segmental duct
LM	left medial segmental duct
LL	left lateral segmental duct

Intrahepatic ducts and segments of liver

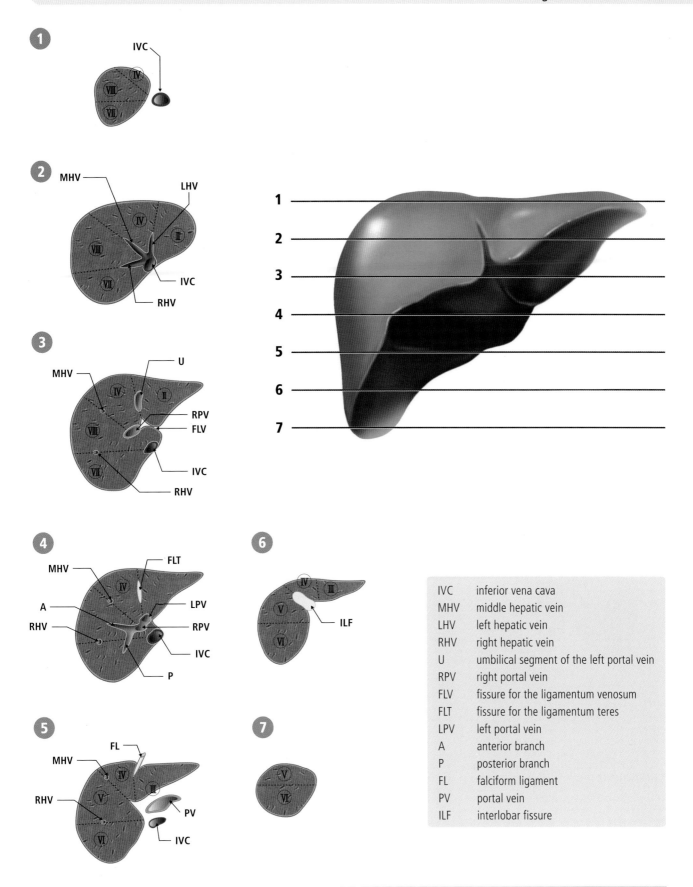

IVC	inferior vena cava
MHV	middle hepatic vein
LHV	left hepatic vein
RHV	right hepatic vein
U	umbilical segment of the left portal vein
RPV	right portal vein
FLV	fissure for the ligamentum venosum
FLT	fissure for the ligamentum teres
LPV	left portal vein
A	anterior branch
P	posterior branch
FL	falciform ligament
PV	portal vein
ILF	interlobar fissure

Segmental anatomy of liver in the transaxial plane at different levels through the liver

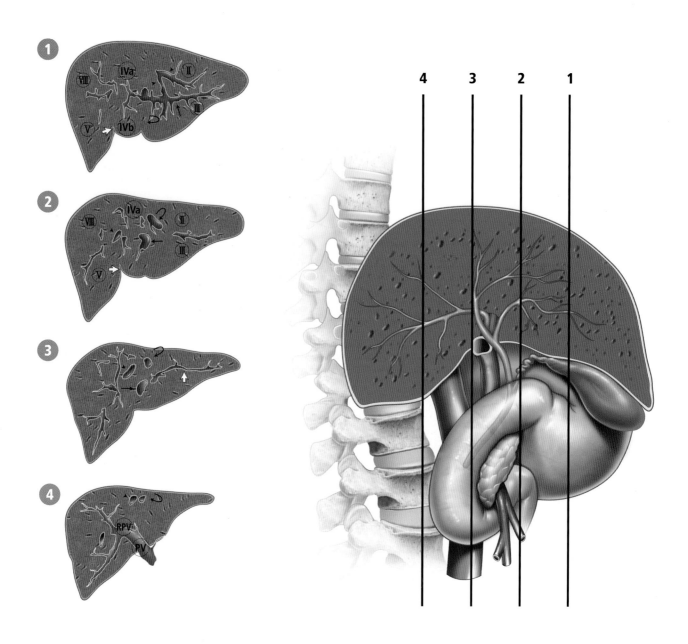

Segmental and venous anatomy of liver in the coronal plane from anterior to posterior

1) Arrow, left lateral portal vein branch to segment III. Arrowheads, left hepatic vein branches draining segments II and III. Curved arrow, fissure for the ligamentum teres. Open arrow, interlobar fissure (gallbladder fossa).

2) Arrow, umbilical segment of the left portal vein. Curved arrow, left hepatic vein. Arrowhead, middle hepatic vein. Open arrow, interlobar fissure (gallbladder fossa).

3) Arrow, umbilical segment of the left portal vein. Curved arrow, left hepatic vein. Arrowhead, middle hepatic vein. Open arrow, left lateral portal vein branch to segment II.

4) Curved arrow, left hepatic vein. Arrowhead, middle hepatic vein. PV, main portal vein. RPV, right portal vein.

03 Artery and vein of pancreaticobiliary system

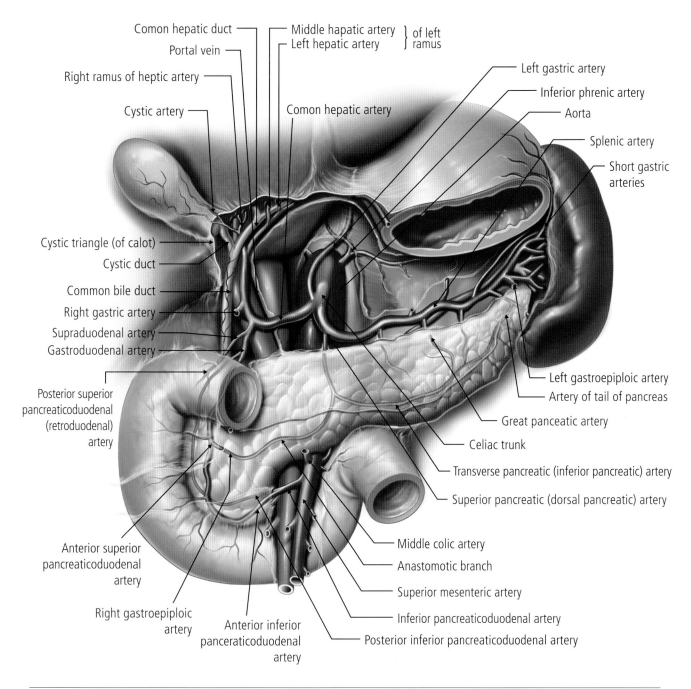

Comon hepatic duct
Middle hapatic artery ⎱ of left
Left hepatic artery ⎰ ramus
Portal vein
Left gastric artery
Right ramus of heptic artery
Inferior phrenic artery
Comon hepatic artery
Aorta
Cystic artery
Splenic artery
Short gastric arteries
Cystic triangle (of calot)
Cystic duct
Common bile duct
Right gastric artery
Supraduodenal artery
Gastroduodenal artery
Left gastroepiploic artery
Artery of tail of pancreas
Posterior superior pancreaticoduodenal (retroduodenal) artery
Great panceatic artery
Celiac trunk
Transverse pancreatic (inferior pancreatic) artery
Superior pancreatic (dorsal pancreatic) artery
Middle colic artery
Anastomotic branch
Anterior superior pancreaticoduodenal artery
Superior mesenteric artery
Right gastroepiploic artery
Inferior pancreaticoduodenal artery
Anterior inferior pancreaticoduodenal artery
Posterior inferior pancreaticoduodenal artery

Artery and vein of pancreaticobiliary system, anterior view

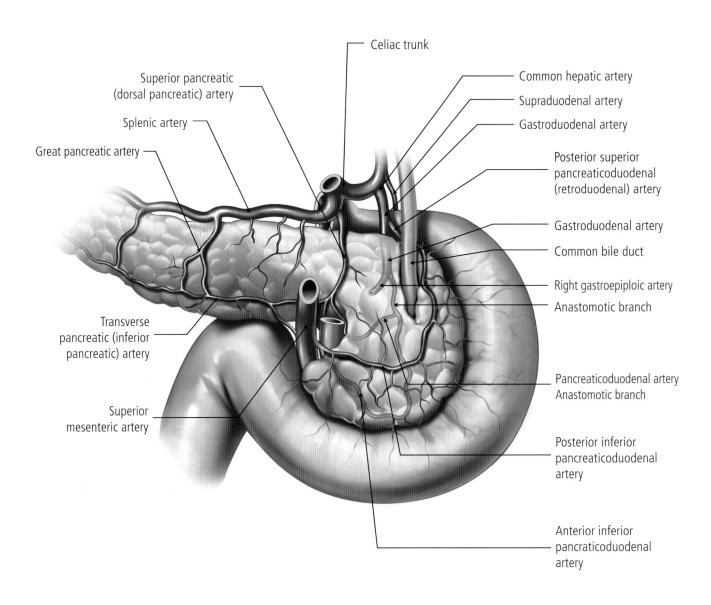

Celiac trunk

Superior pancreatic
(dorsal pancreatic) artery

Splenic artery

Great pancreatic artery

Transverse
pancreatic (inferior
pancreatic) artery

Superior
mesenteric artery

Common hepatic artery

Supraduodenal artery

Gastroduodenal artery

Posterior superior
pancreaticoduodenal
(retroduodenal) artery

Gastroduodenal artery

Common bile duct

Right gastroepiploic artery

Anastomotic branch

Pancreaticoduodenal artery
Anastomotic branch

Posterior inferior
pancreaticoduodenal
artery

Anterior inferior
pancraticoduodenal
artery

Artery and vein of pancreaticobiliary system, posterior view

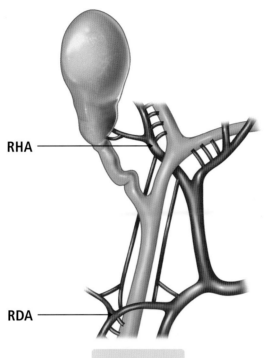

RHA

RDA

RHA	right hepatic artery
RDA	retroduodenal artery
RPA	retroportal artery

Anterior view

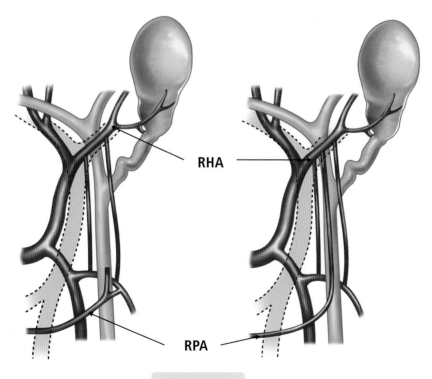

RHA

RPA

Posterior view

Blood supply to extrahepatic duct

04 Biliary tract

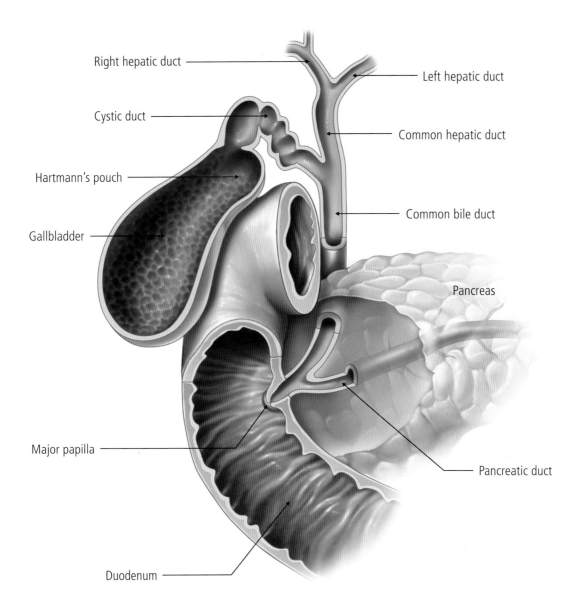

Right hepatic duct

Cystic duct

Hartmann's pouch

Gallbladder

Left hepatic duct

Common hepatic duct

Common bile duct

Pancreas

Major papilla

Pancreatic duct

Duodenum

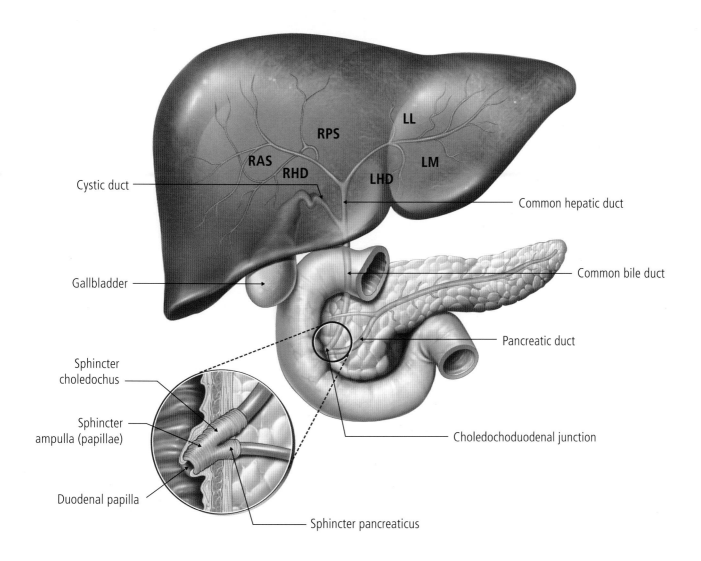

Cystic duct

RAS
RPS
RHD
LHD
LL
LM

Common hepatic duct

Gallbladder

Common bile duct

Pancreatic duct

Sphincter
choledochus

Sphincter
ampulla (papillae)

Choledochoduodenal junction

Duodenal papilla

Sphincter pancreaticus

RHD	right hepatic duct
LHD	left hepatic duct
RAS	right anterior segmental duct
RPS	right posterior segmental duct
LL	left lateral segmental duct
LM	left medial segmental duct

Frontal view of normal biliary tract

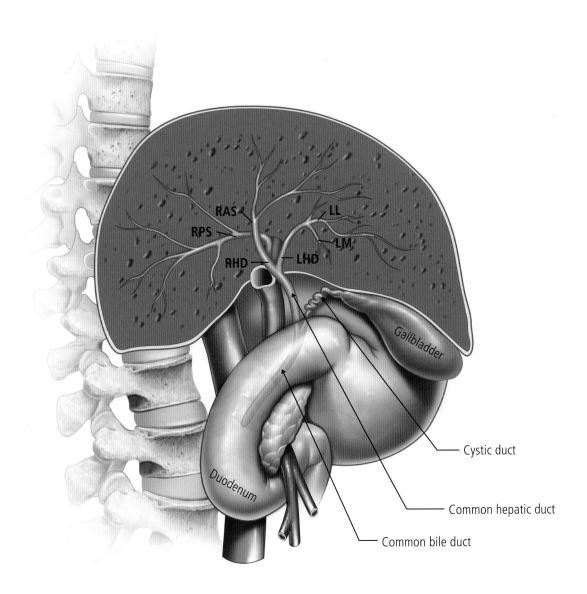

RHD	right hepatic duct
LHD	left hepatic duct
RAS	right anterior segmental duct
RPS	right posterior segmental duct
LL	left lateral segmental duct
LM	left medial segmental duct

Lateral view of normal biliary tract

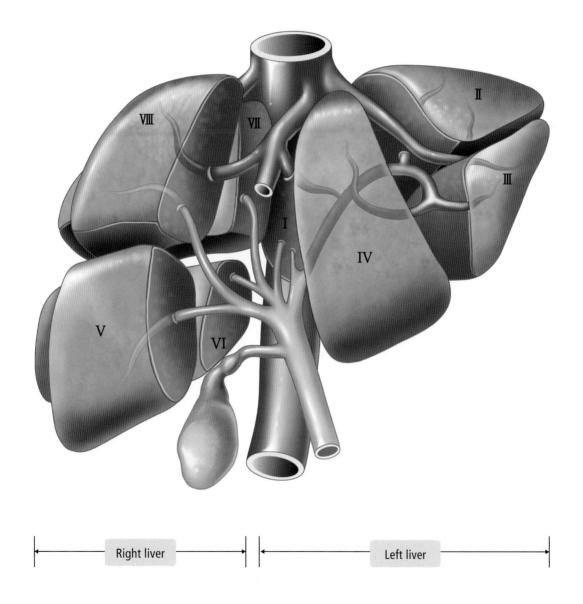

Biliary drainage of two functional hemilivers

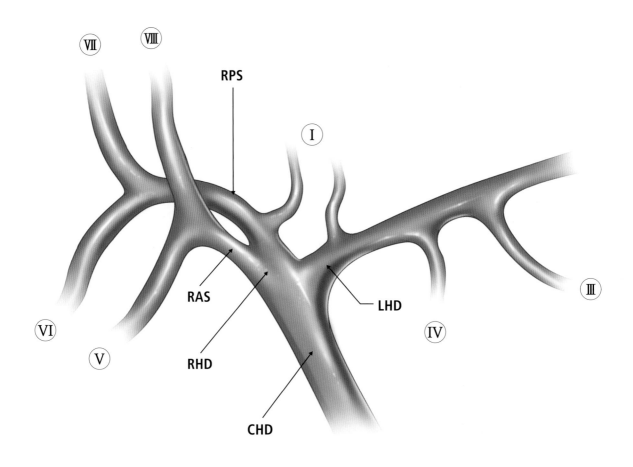

CHD	common hepatic duct
RHD	right hepatic duct
LHD	left hepatic duct
RAS	right anterior segmental duct
RPS	right posterior segmental duct

Standard anatomy of intrahepatic ducts

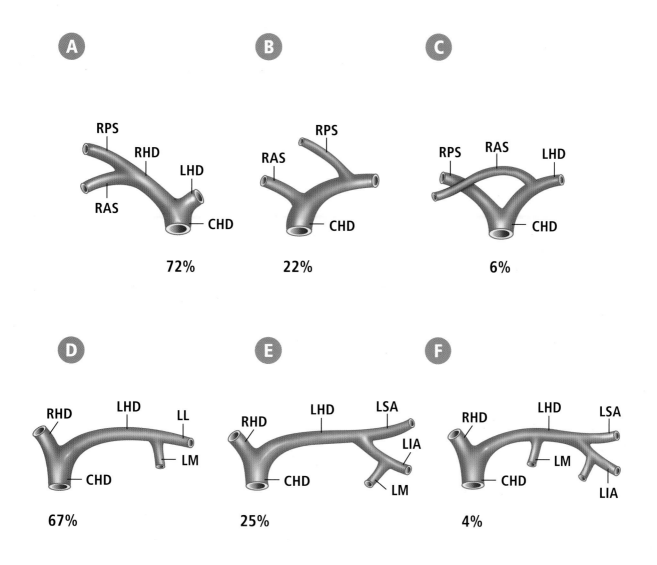

A-C	variations related to the right lobe
D-F	variations related to the left lobe
RAS	right anterior segmental duct
RPS	right posterior segmental duct
LM	left medial segmental duct
LL	left lateral segmental duct
RHD	right hepatic duct
LHD	left hepatic duct
LIA	lateral inferior area duct
LSA	lateral superior area duct
CHD	common hepatic duct

Variations of intrahepatic ducts

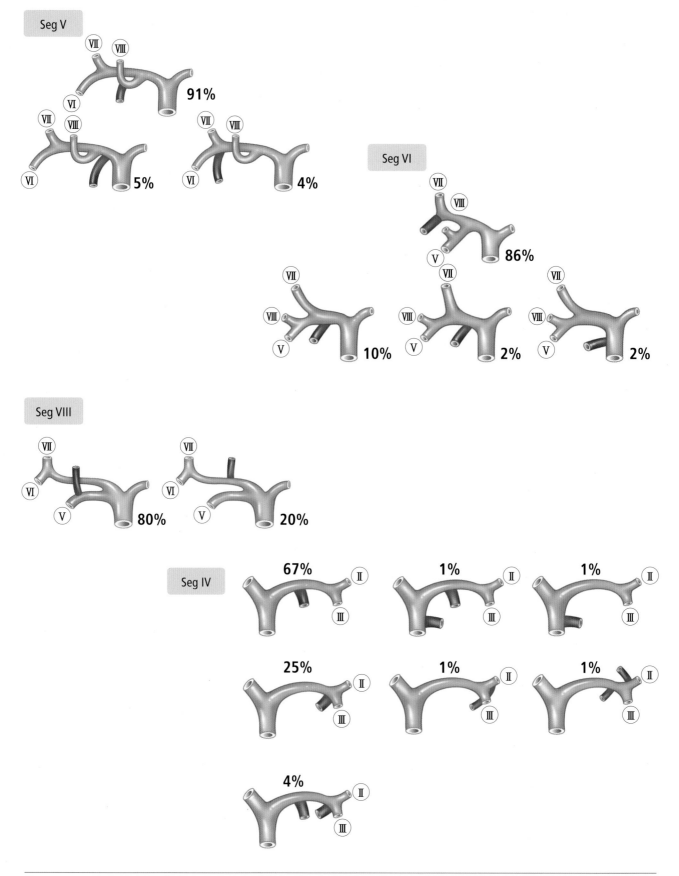

Common variations of the segmental intrahepatic ducts

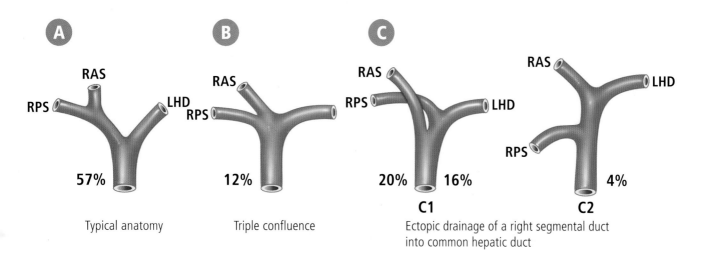

A RAS RPS LHD

57%

Typical anatomy

B RAS RPS LHD

12%

Triple confluence

C RAS RPS LHD

20%   16%

C1

RAS LHD RPS

4%

C2

Ectopic drainage of a right segmental duct
into common hepatic duct

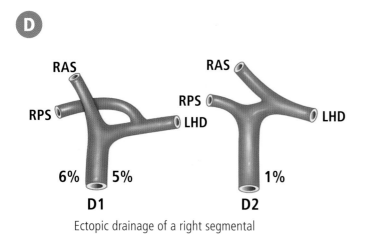

D RAS RPS LHD

6%   5%

D1

RAS RPS LHD

1%

D2

Ectopic drainage of a right segmental
duct into left hepatic duct

RAS	right anterior segmental duct
RPS	right posterior segmental duct
LHD	left hepatic duct

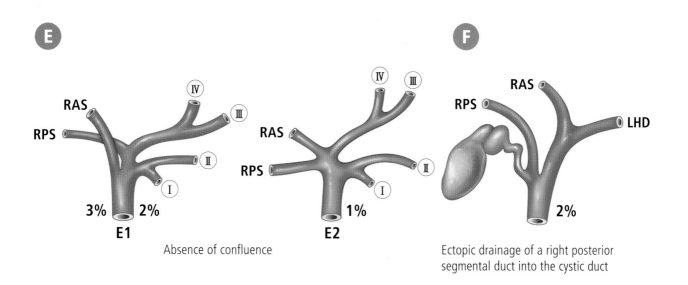

E RAS RPS ⅣⅢ Ⅱ Ⅰ

3%   2%

E1

RAS RPS ⅣⅢ Ⅱ Ⅰ

1%

E2

Absence of confluence

F RAS RPS LHD

2%

Ectopic drainage of a right posterior
segmental duct into the cystic duct

Common variations of biliary confluence anatomy

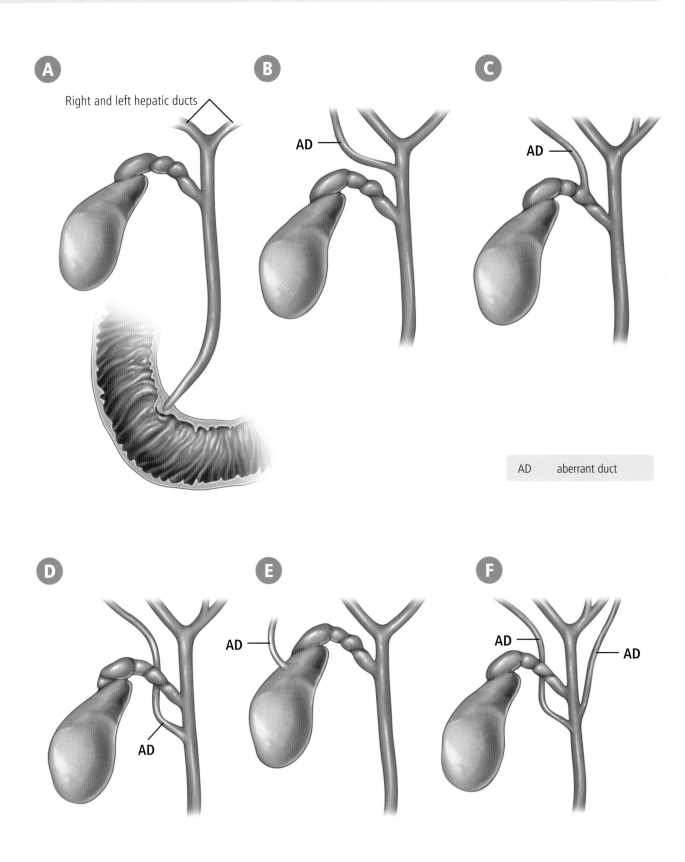

Anomalous variations of hepatic ducts

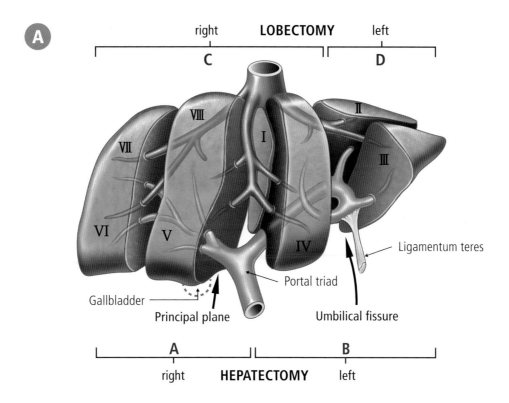

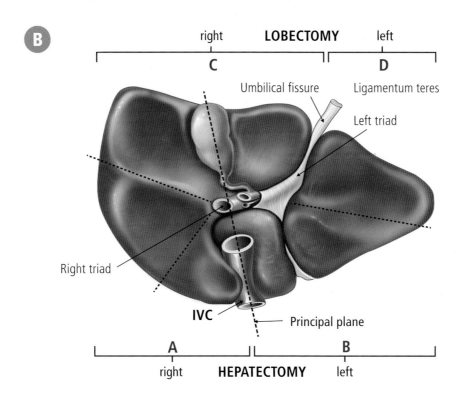

Surgical anatomy of the liver

A) Enlarged view to show the sectors (separated by the major hepatic veins) and the segmental structure of the liver. Each segment is supplied by a portal triad; the left portal pedicle traverses beneath segment IV to the umbilical fissure; the umbilical portion of the pedicle curves ventrally and caudally in the umbilical fissure. The blood supply to segment IV is recurrent as feedback vessels.

B) Inferior surface of the liver; segment VIII is not seen because it lies superiorly. The anatomic division into right and left lobes by the umbilical fissure and into a right and left liver in the principal plane, along the principal scissura, is evident. IVC, inferior vena cava.

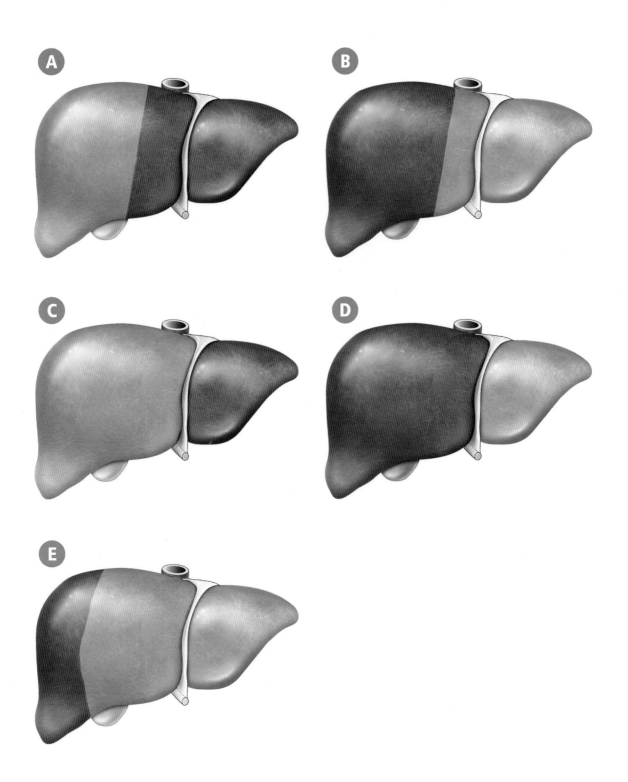

Commonly performed major hepatic resections

A) Right hepatectomy. B) Left hepatectomy. C) Right lobectomy. D) Left lobectomy. E) Extended left hepatectomy.

05 Pancreas

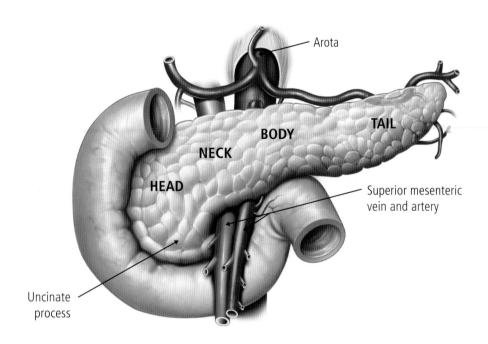

Arota

BODY

NECK

TAIL

HEAD

Superior mesenteric
vein and artery

Uncinate
process

UNCINATE PROCESS

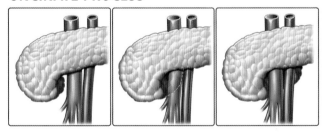

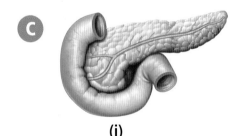

(i)

POSITION OF THE COMMON BILE DUCT

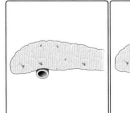

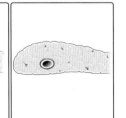

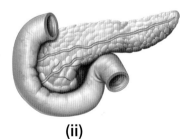

(ii)

A) Extent of uncinate process. B) Position of common bile duct relative to the pancreas.
C) (i) Normal anatomy, (ii) Pancreas divisum.

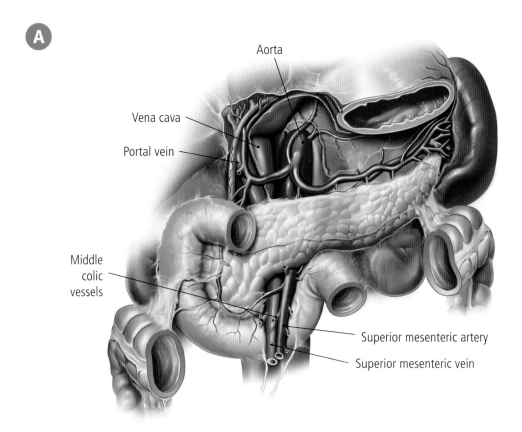

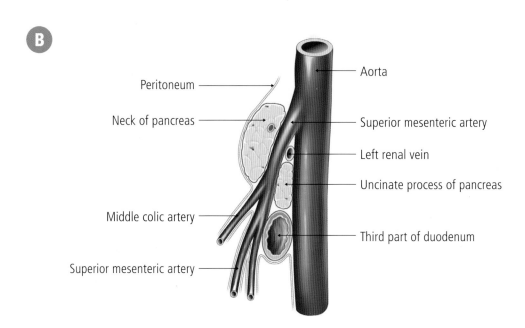

A) Anterior view of the pancreas.
B) Relationship of the pancreatic neck and uncinate process to the aorta and superior mesenteric artery.

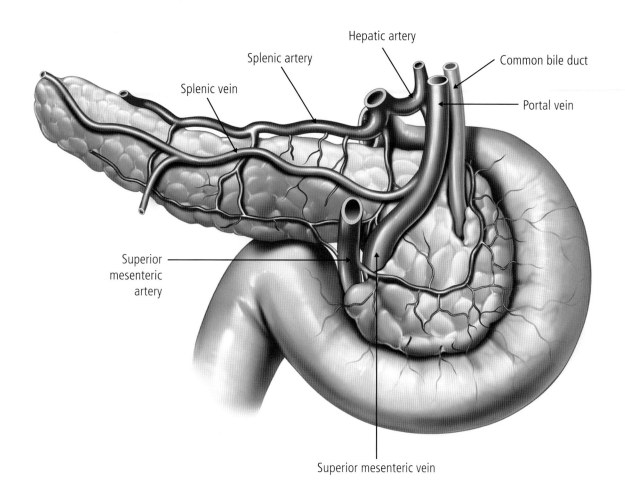

Hepatic artery

Splenic artery

Common bile duct

Splenic vein

Portal vein

Superior
mesenteric
artery

Superior mesenteric vein

Posterior view of the pancreas

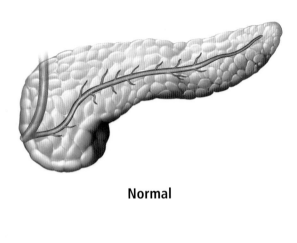

Normal

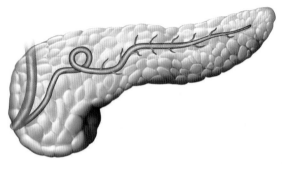

Loop
(Ansa pancreatica)

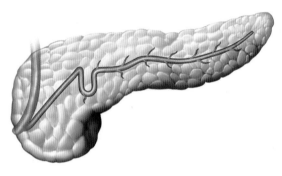

N configuration

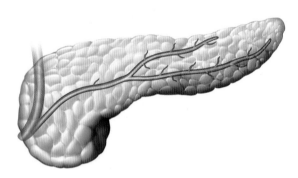

Bifurcation

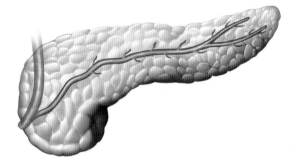

Bifurcation

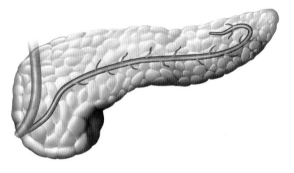

Angulation

Pancreatic ductal system and its variations

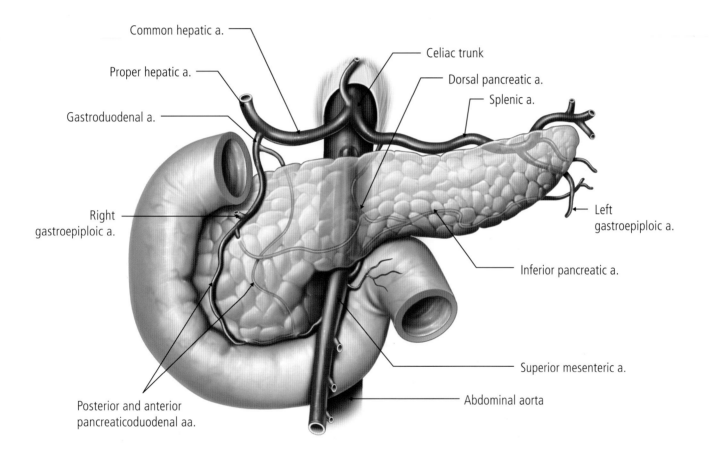

Common hepatic a.

Proper hepatic a.

Gastroduodenal a.

Right
gastroepiploic a.

Posterior and anterior
pancreaticoduodenal aa.

Celiac trunk

Dorsal pancreatic a.

Splenic a.

Left
gastroepiploic a.

Inferior pancreatic a.

Superior mesenteric a.

Abdominal aorta

Arterial supply of pancreas, anterior view (1)

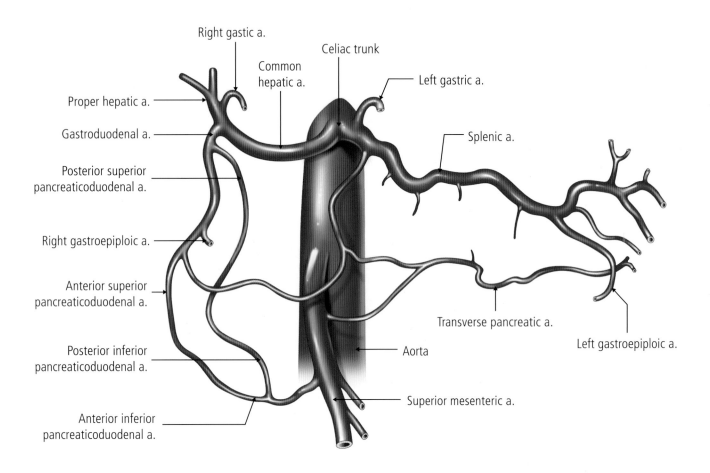

Arterial supply of pancreas, anterior view (2)

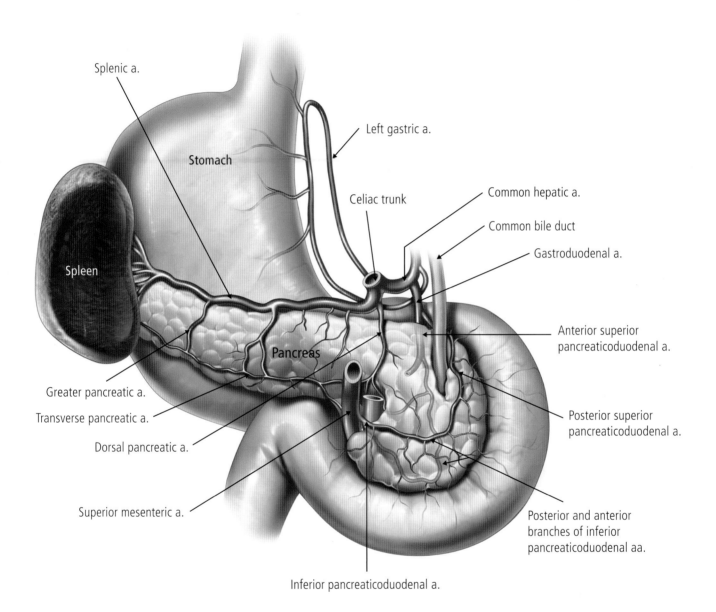

Splenic a.

Left gastric a.

Stomach

Celiac trunk

Common hepatic a.

Common bile duct

Gastroduodenal a.

Spleen

Pancreas

Anterior superior
pancreaticoduodenal a.

Greater pancreatic a.

Transverse pancreatic a.

Dorsal pancreatic a.

Posterior superior
pancreaticoduodenal a.

Superior mesenteric a.

Posterior and anterior
branches of inferior
pancreaticoduodenal aa.

Inferior pancreaticoduodenal a.

Arterial supply of pancreas, posterior view

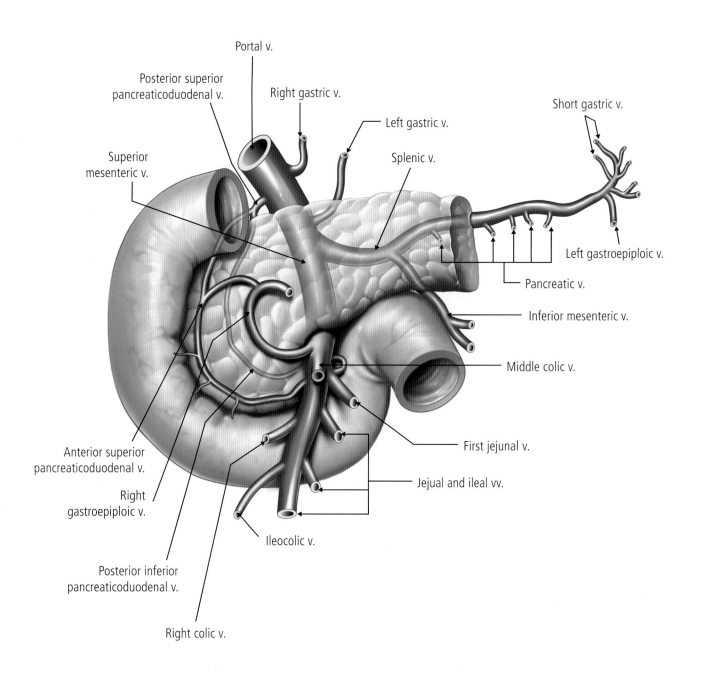

Portal v.

Posterior superior
pancreaticoduodenal v.

Right gastric v.

Left gastric v.

Short gastric v.

Superior
mesenteric v.

Splenic v.

Left gastroepiploic v.

Pancreatic v.

Inferior mesenteric v.

Middle colic v.

Anterior superior
pancreaticoduodenal v.

First jejunal v.

Right
gastroepiploic v.

Jejual and ileal vv.

Posterior inferior
pancreaticoduodenal v.

Ileocolic v.

Right colic v.

Venous drainage of pancreas

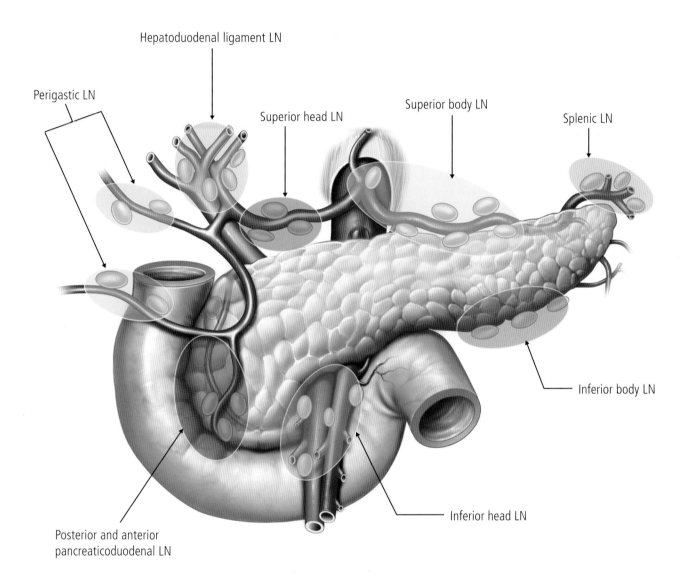

Hepatoduodenal ligament LN

Perigastic LN

Superior head LN

Superior body LN

Splenic LN

Inferior body LN

Inferior head LN

Posterior and anterior
pancreaticoduodenal LN

LN   lymph node

Lymphatic drainage of pancreas

06 Gallbladder and cystic duct

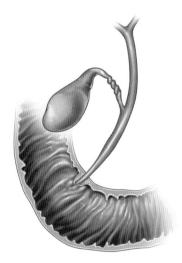

Normal

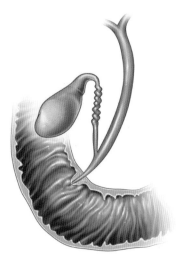

Low union with
extrahepatic bile duct

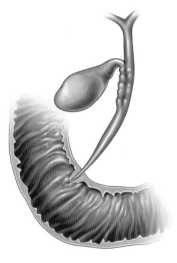

Parallel course and
common sheath with
extrahepatic bile duct

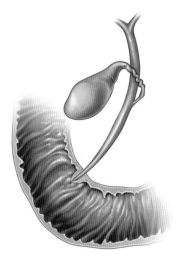

Anterior spiral to left
side of extrahepatic bile duct

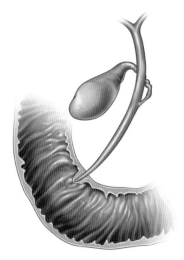

Posterior spiral to left
side of extrahepatic bile duct

Variations of cystic duct insertion (1)

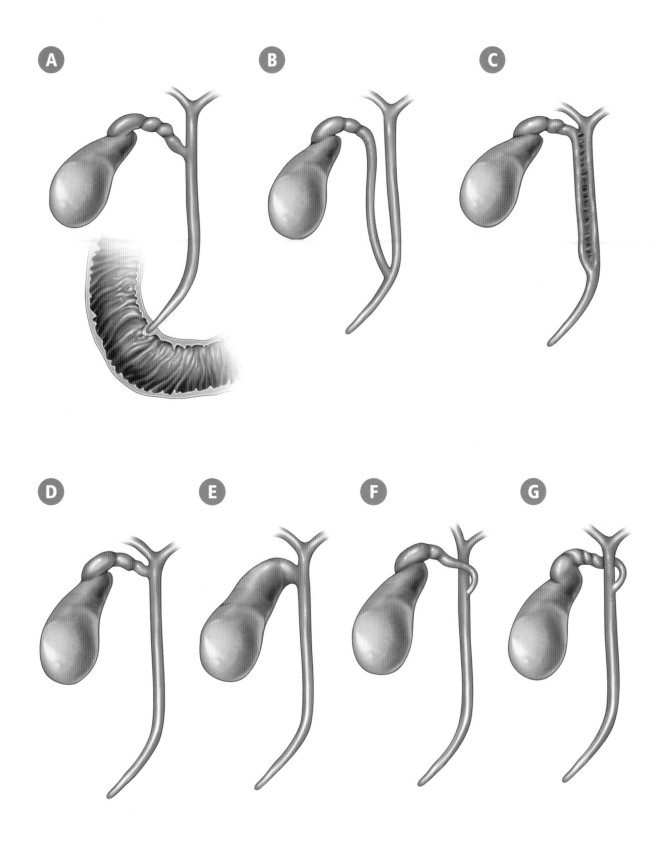

Variations of cystic duct insertion (2)

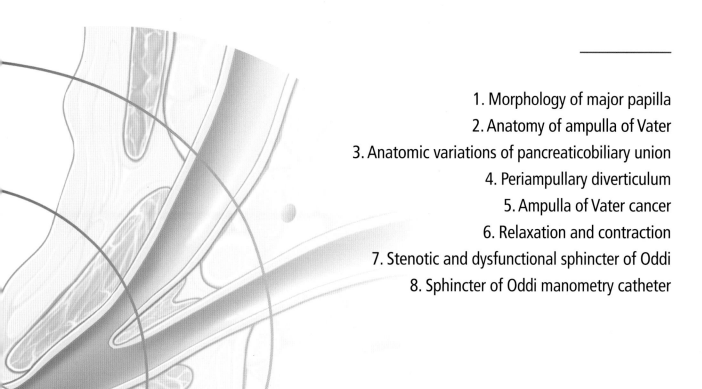

PART

II

Ampulla of Vater

01 Morphology of major papilla

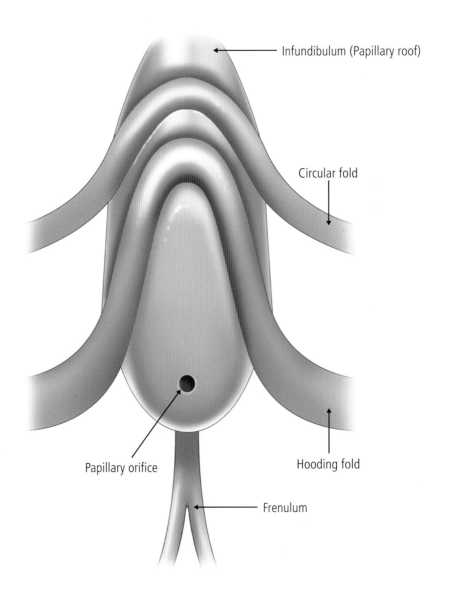

Infundibulum (Papillary roof)

Circular fold

Hooding fold

Papillary orifice

Frenulum

Gross morphology of major papilla

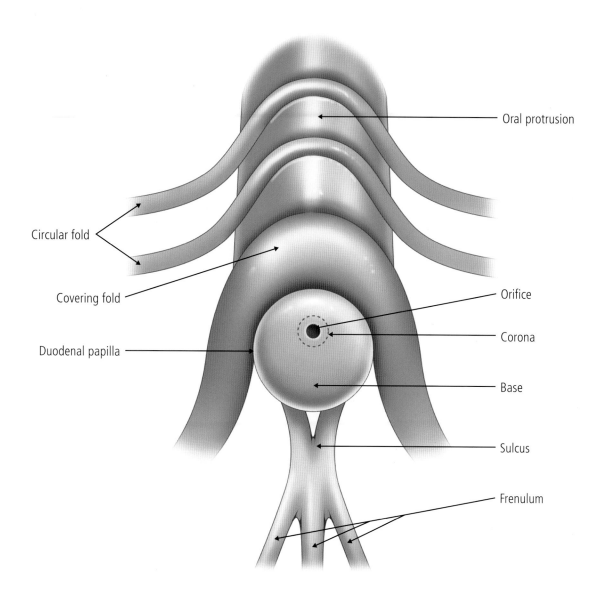

Oral protrusion

Circular fold

Covering fold

Duodenal papilla

Orifice

Corona

Base

Sulcus

Frenulum

External morphology of major papilla

02 Anatomy of ampulla of Vater

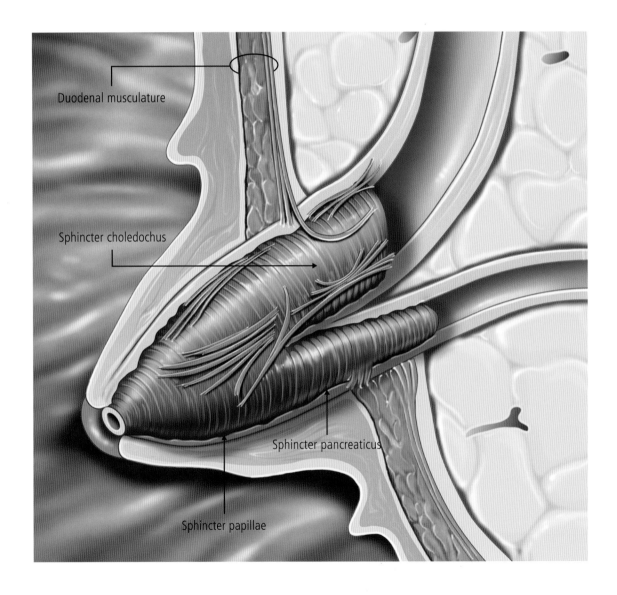

Duodenal musculature

Sphincter choledochus

Sphincter pancreaticus

Sphincter papillae

Anatomical structure of the sphincter of Oddi

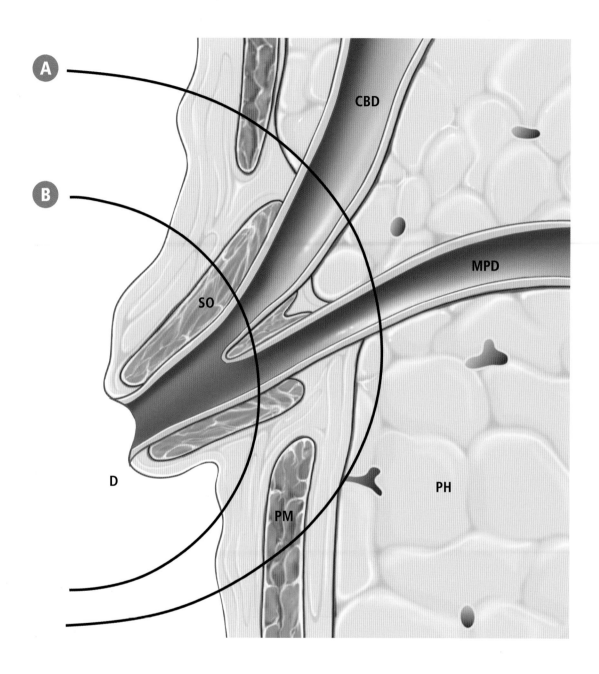

CBD	common bile duct	MPD	main pancreatic duct
SO	sphincter of Oddi	PM	proper muscle of duodenum
D	duodenal lumen	PH	pancreas head

A) Surgical ampullectomy line
B) Endoscopic papillectomy line

03 Anatomic variations of pancreaticobiliary union

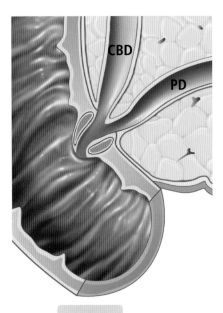

| CBD | common bile duct |
| PD | pancreatic duct |

Y type

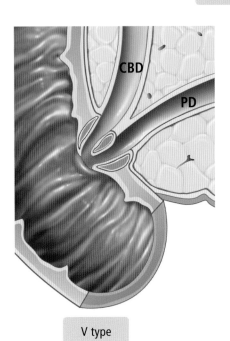

V type

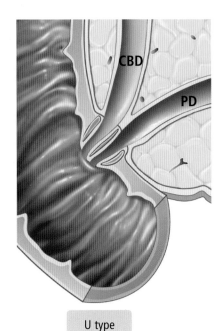

U type

Anatomic variations of pancreaticobiliary duct union

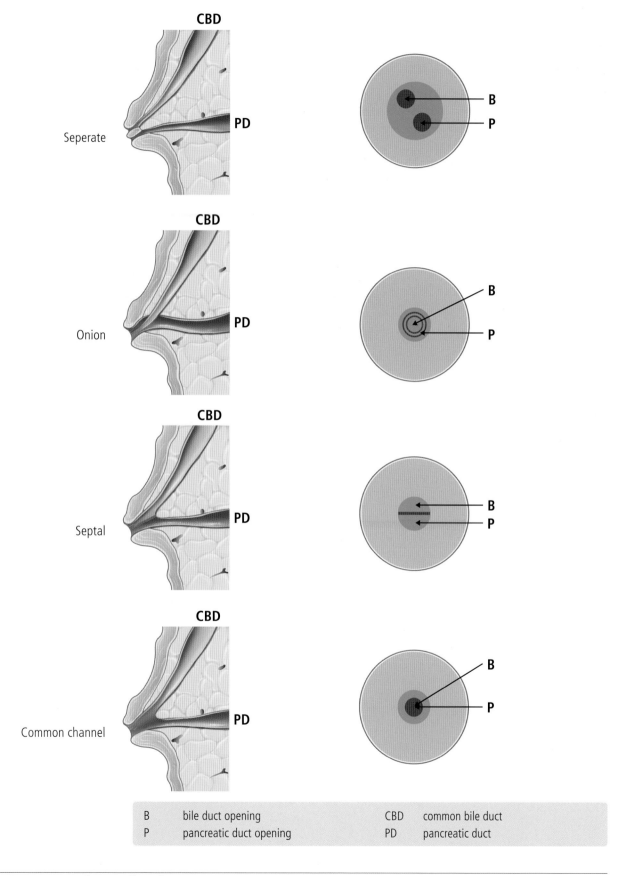

| B | bile duct opening | CBD | common bile duct |
| P | pancreatic duct opening | PD | pancreatic duct |

Opening types of ampulla of Vater

04 Periampullary diverticulum

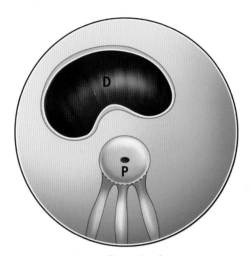

Extradiverticulum

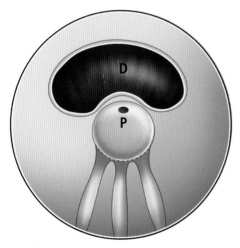

Juxtadiverticulum

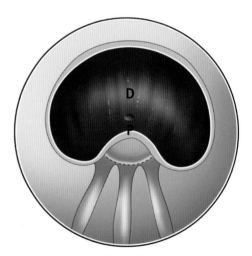

Intradiverticulum

D	diverticulum
P	papilla

Types of periampullary diverticulum

05 Ampulla of Vater cancer

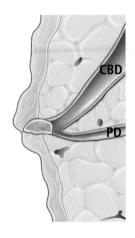

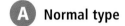

A Normal type

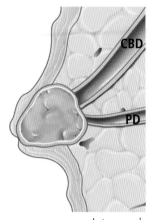

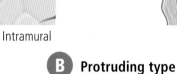

Intramural   Exposed

B Protruding type

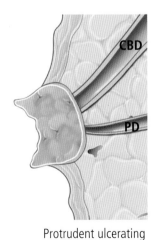

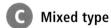

Protrudent ulcerating

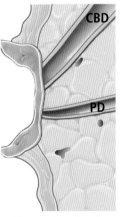

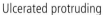

Ulcerated protruding

C Mixed type

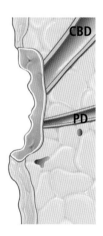

D Ulcerating type

| CBD | common bile duct |
| PD | pancreatic duct |

Morphologic classification of ampulla of Vater cancer

06 Relaxation and contraction

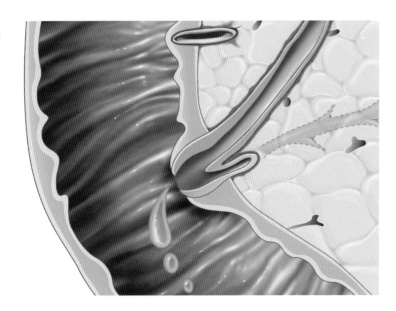

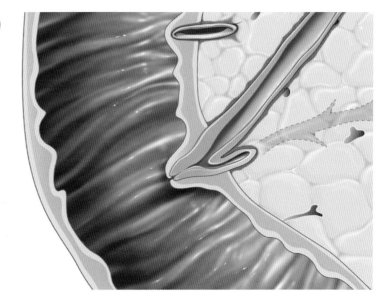

A) Relaxation
B) Contraction

07 Stenotic and dysfunctional sphincter of Oddi

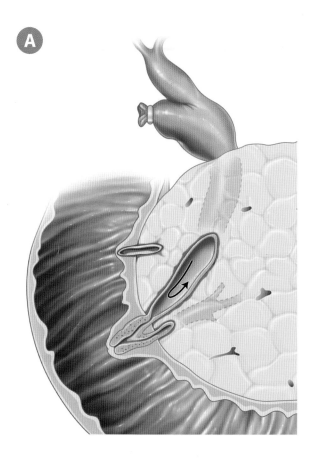

SO	sphincter of Oddi

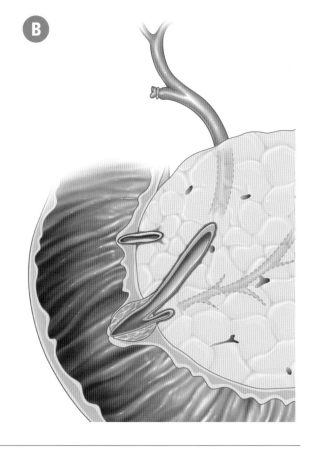

A) Stenotic SO
B) Dysfunctional SO

08 Sphincter of Oddi manometry catheter

❶ Lehman catheter

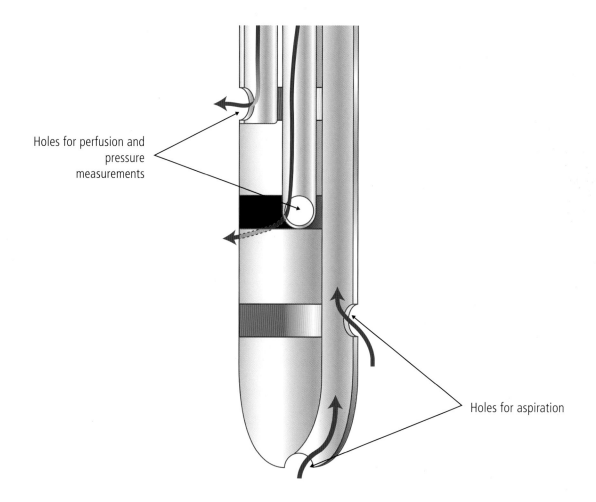

Holes for perfusion and pressure measurements

Holes for aspiration

❷ Sphinter of Oddi manometry (SOM)

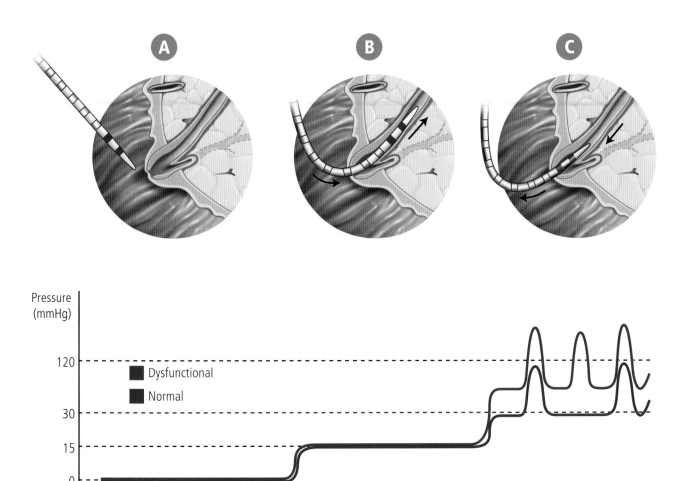

A) Baseline calibration in duodenum
B) Insertion of SOM catheter into common bile duct
C) Pulling SOM catheter back from common bile duct

Suggested abnormal values of SOM

Basal sphincter pressure	> 40 mmHg
Basal ductal pressure	> 13 mmHg
Phasic contractions Amplitude Duration Frequency	 > 220 mmHg > 8 sec > 10/min

III

Biliary Tract

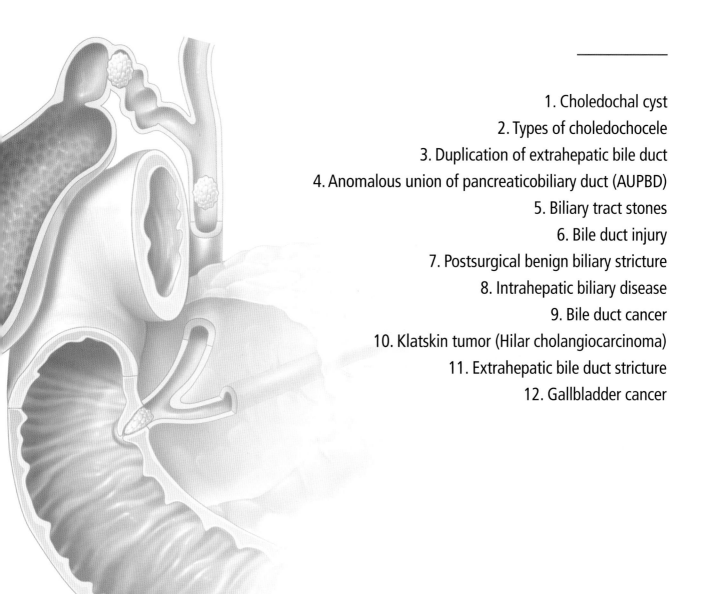

01 Choledochal cyst

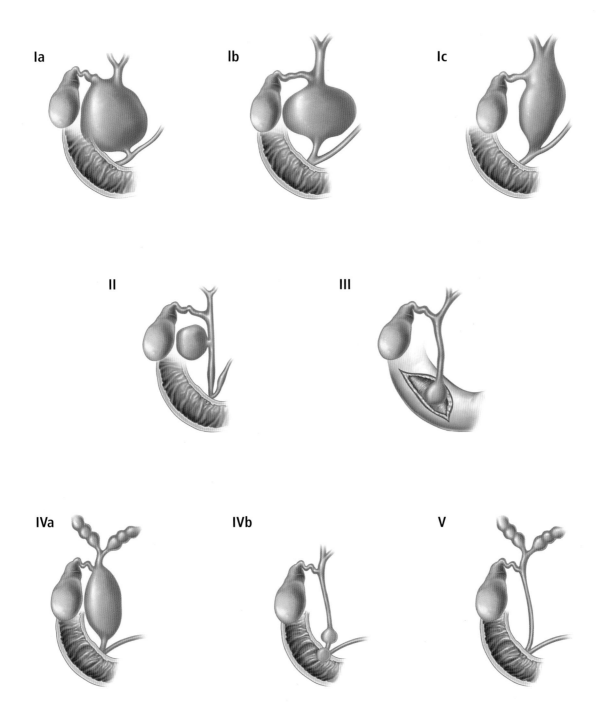

Todani's classification of choledochal cysts

02 Types of choledochocele

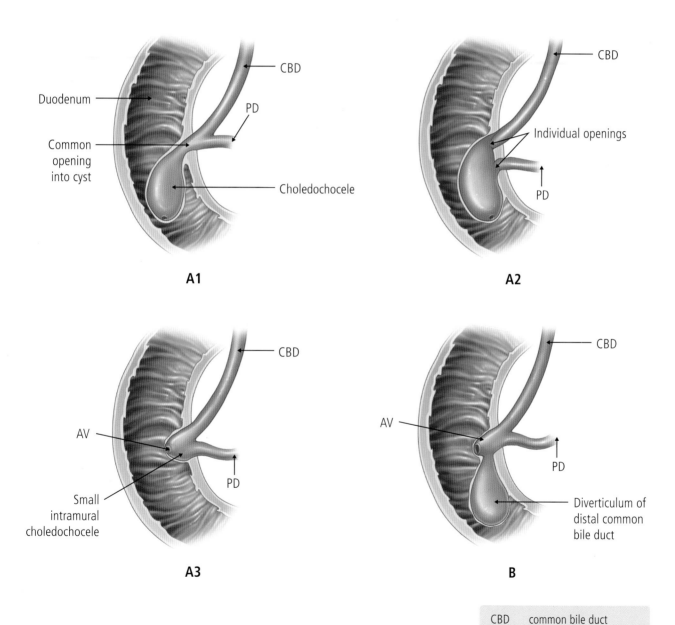

A1

A2

A3

B

CBD	common bile duct
PD	pancreatic duct
AV	ampulla of Vater

Classification of choledochoceles

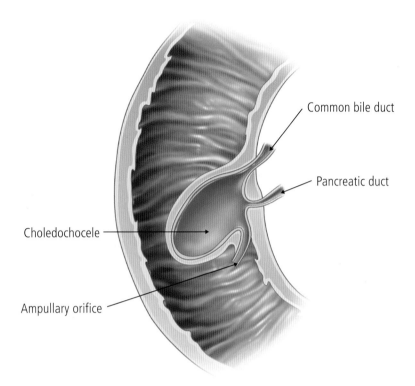

Common bile duct

Pancreatic duct

Choledochocele

Ampullary orifice

Type 1

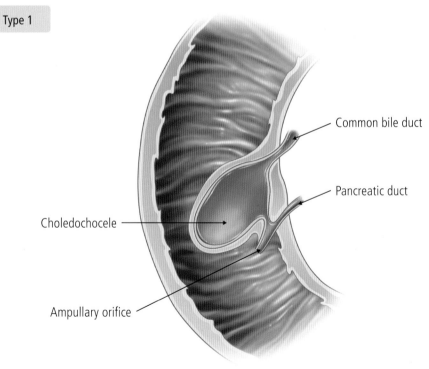

Common bile duct

Pancreatic duct

Choledochocele

Ampullary orifice

Type 2

Classification of choledochoceles

03 Duplication of extrahepatic bile duct

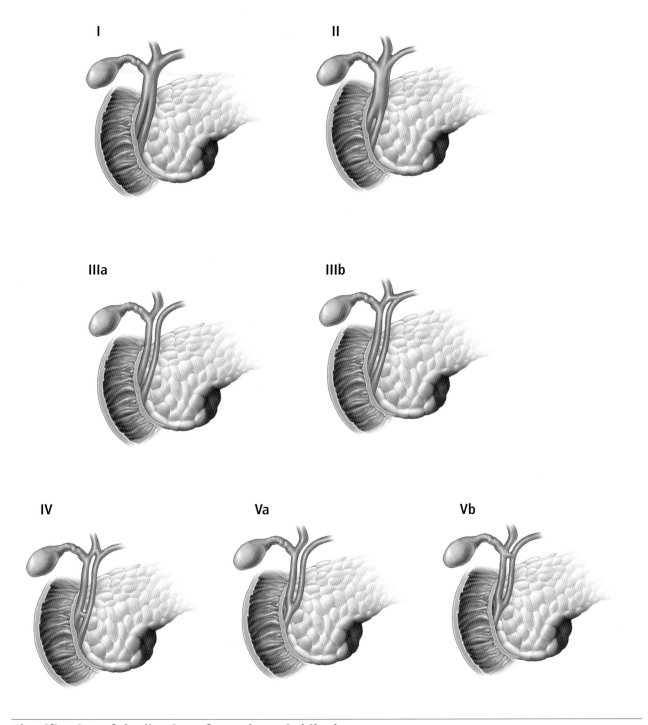

Classification of duplication of extrahepatic bile duct

04 Anomalous union of pancreaticobiliary duct (AUPBD)

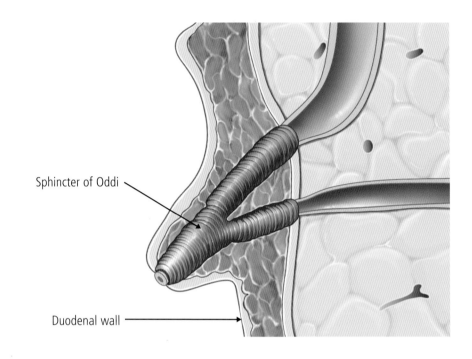

Normal union

Sphincter of Oddi

Duodenal wall

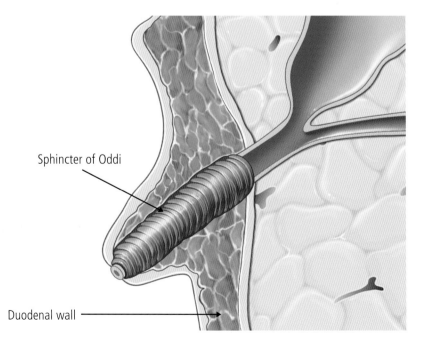

Abnormal union

Sphincter of Oddi

Duodenal wall

Anatomical relationship of sphincter and duodenal wall

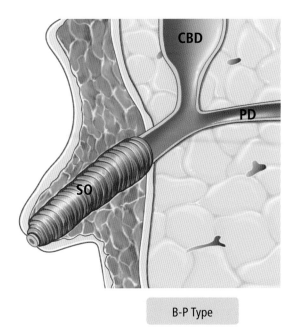

B-P Type

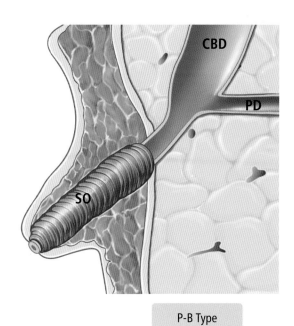

P-B Type

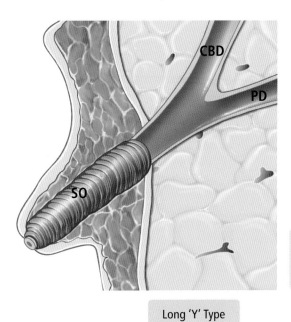

Long 'Y' Type

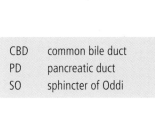

CBD	common bile duct
PD	pancreatic duct
SO	sphincter of Oddi

Three types of AUPBD

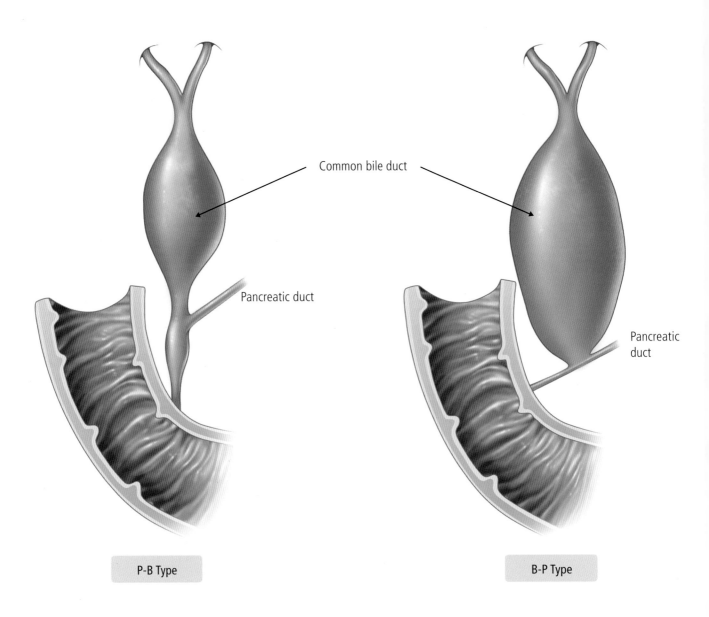

Common bile duct

Pancreatic duct

Pancreatic duct

P-B Type

B-P Type

Kimura's classification of AUPBD

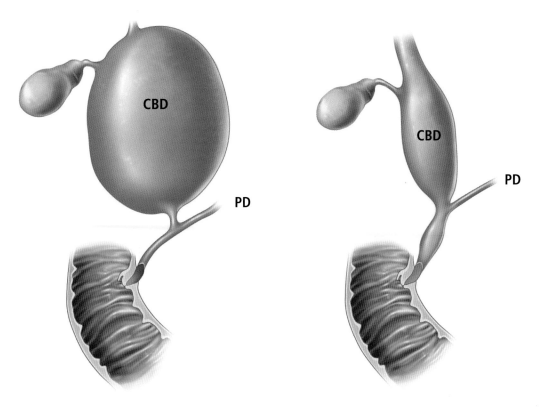

Type A : non-dilated common channel

Type B : dilated common channel

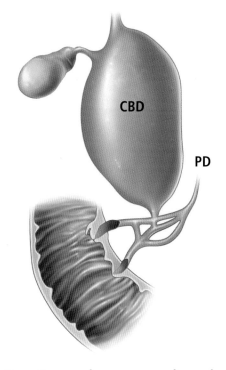

Type C : complex common channel

| CBD | common bile duct |
| PD | pancreatic duct |

Todani's classification of AUPBD

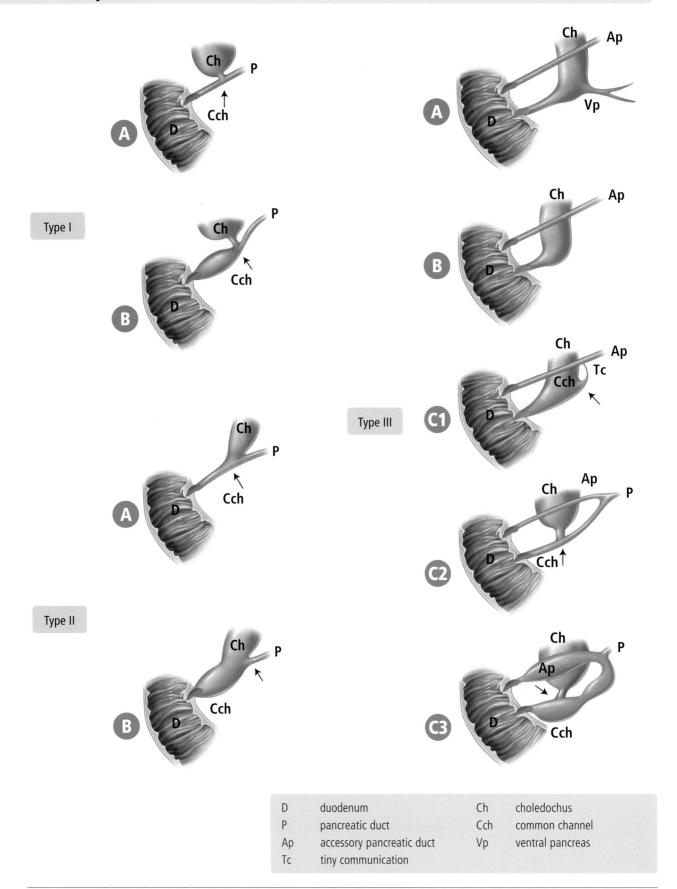

D	duodenum	Ch	choledochus
P	pancreatic duct	Cch	common channel
Ap	accessory pancreatic duct	Vp	ventral pancreas
Tc	tiny communication		

Pancreatic ductal system and its variations, Komi classification

05 Biliary tract stones

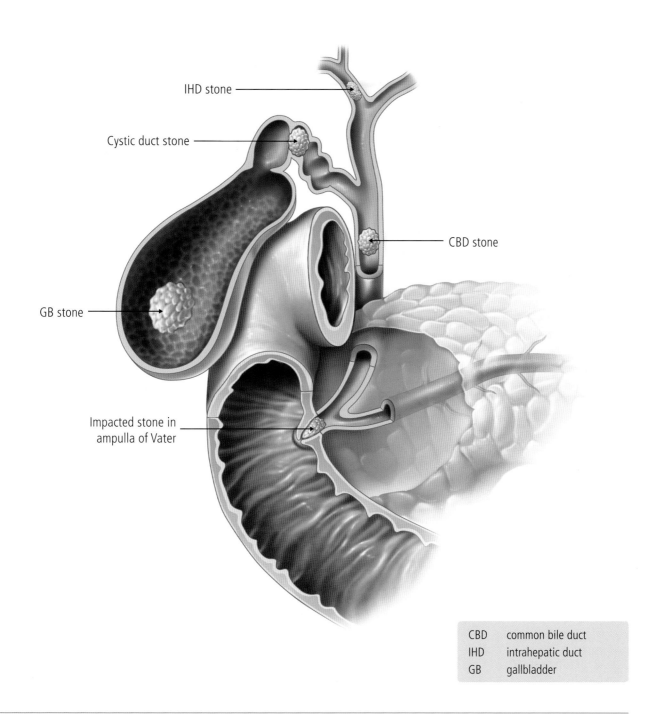

IHD stone

Cystic duct stone

CBD stone

GB stone

Impacted stone in
ampulla of Vater

CBD	common bile duct
IHD	intrahepatic duct
GB	gallbladder

Classification of biliary stones according to location

06 Bile duct injury

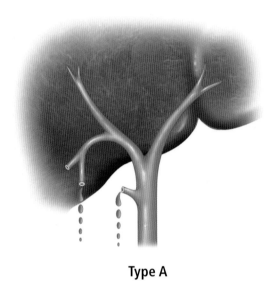

Type A

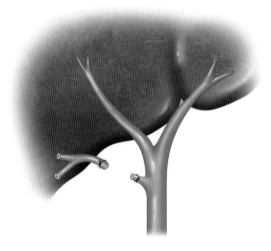

Type B

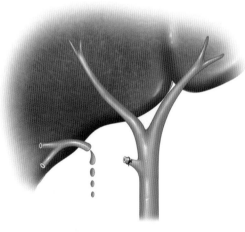

Type C

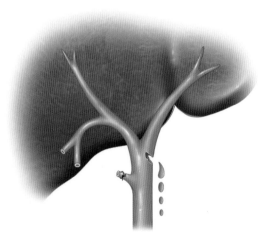

Type D

Classification of bile duct injury following cholecystectomy

07 Postsurgical benign biliary stricture

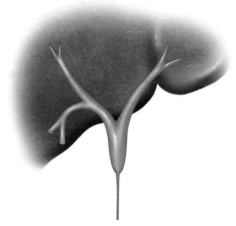

Type I : bifurcation > 2cm

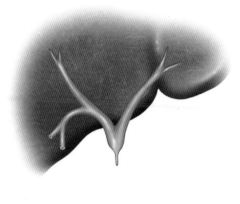

Type II : bifurcation < 2cm

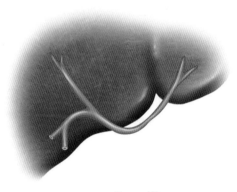

Type III

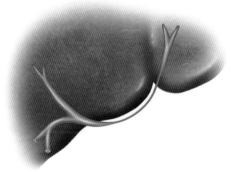

Type IV

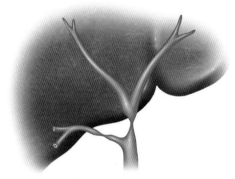

Type V

Bismuth-Lazorthes classification of postsurgical benign biliary strictures

08 Intrahepatic biliary disease

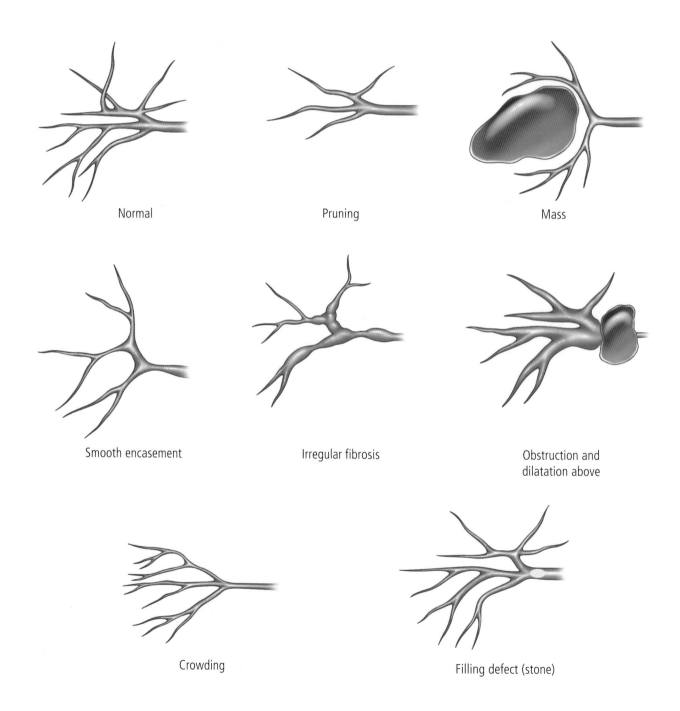

Normal

Pruning

Mass

Smooth encasement

Irregular fibrosis

Obstruction and
dilatation above

Crowding

Filling defect (stone)

Cholangiographic appearances of intrahepatic biliary diseases

09 Bile duct cancer

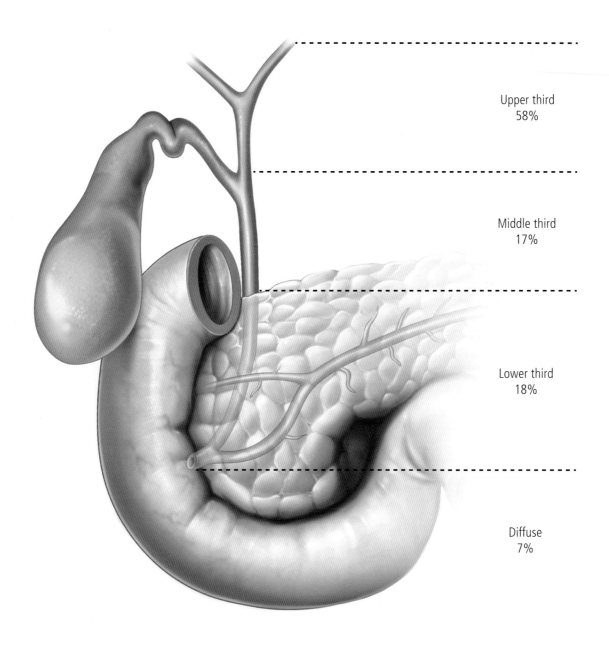

Upper third
58%

Middle third
17%

Lower third
18%

Diffuse
7%

Anatomical distribution of extrahepatic bile duct cancers

Nodular

Papillary

Diffusely
infiltrating

Annular
stricture

**Gross
appearance**

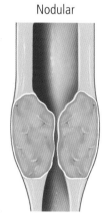 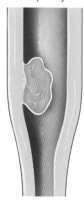 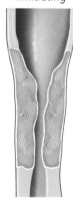 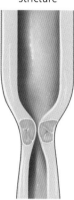

**Cholangiographic
appearance**

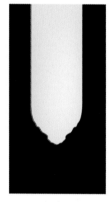 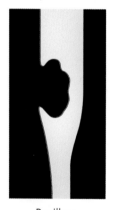 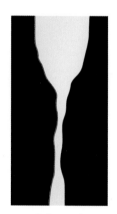 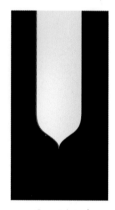

Protuberant

Papillary
protuberant

Sclerosed

Constricted

Cholangiographic appearances of extrahepatic bile duct cancers

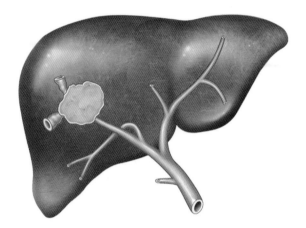

Mass forming type

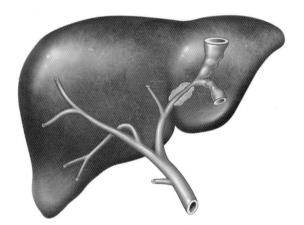

Periductal infiltrative type

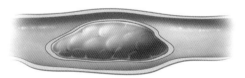

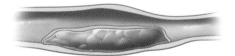

Intraductal growing type

Morphologic types of cholangiocarcinoma

10 Klatskin tumor (Hilar cholangiocarcinoma)

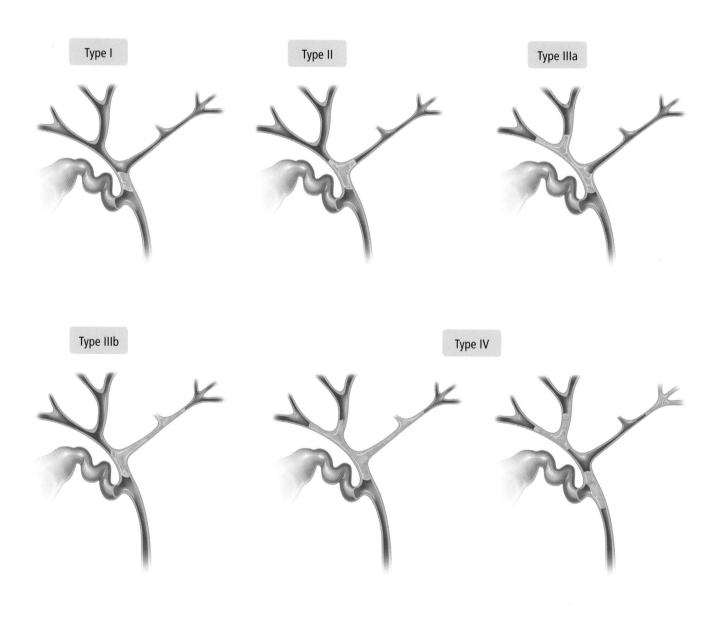

Type I

Type II

Type IIIa

Type IIIb

Type IV

Bismuth classification of Klatskin tumors

11 Extrahepatic bile duct stricture

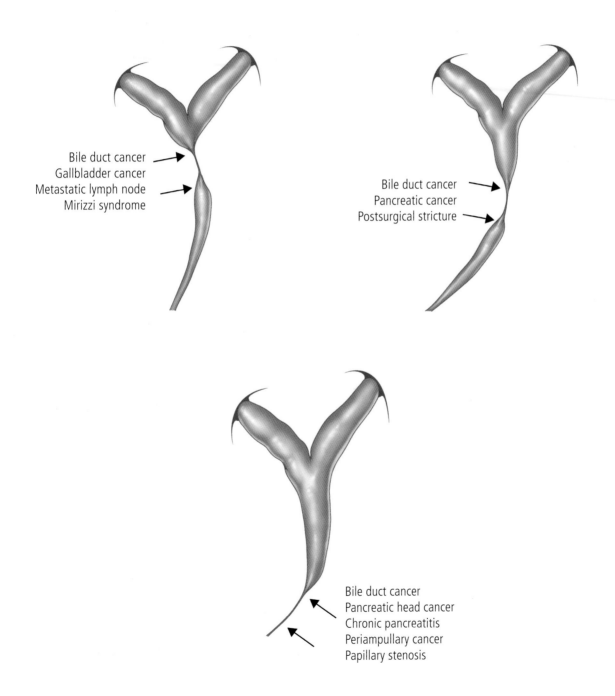

Bile duct cancer
Gallbladder cancer
Metastatic lymph node
Mirizzi syndrome

Bile duct cancer
Pancreatic cancer
Postsurgical stricture

Bile duct cancer
Pancreatic head cancer
Chronic pancreatitis
Periampullary cancer
Papillary stenosis

Differential diagnosis of extrahepatic bile duct stricture

12 / Gallbladder cancer

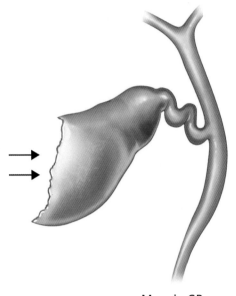

Mass in GB

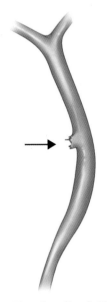

Nonvisualized GB

GB	gallbladder
CHD	common hepatic duct
CBD	common bile duct

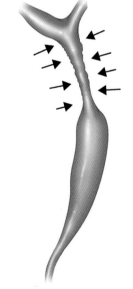

Stricture of CHD or CBD

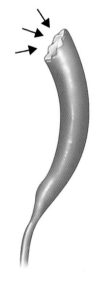

Biliary obstruction

Morphology of gallbladder cancer

IV

Pancreas

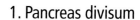

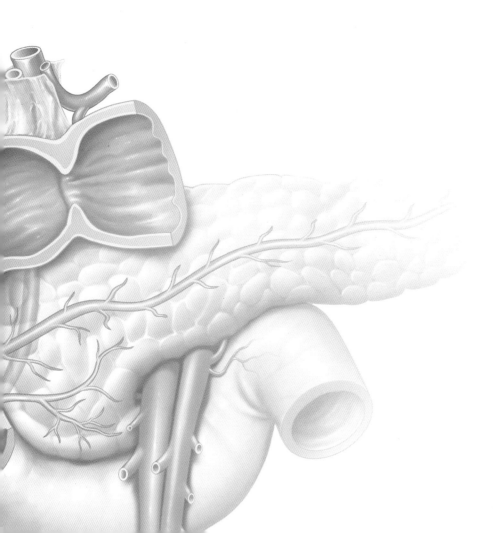

01 Pancreas divisum

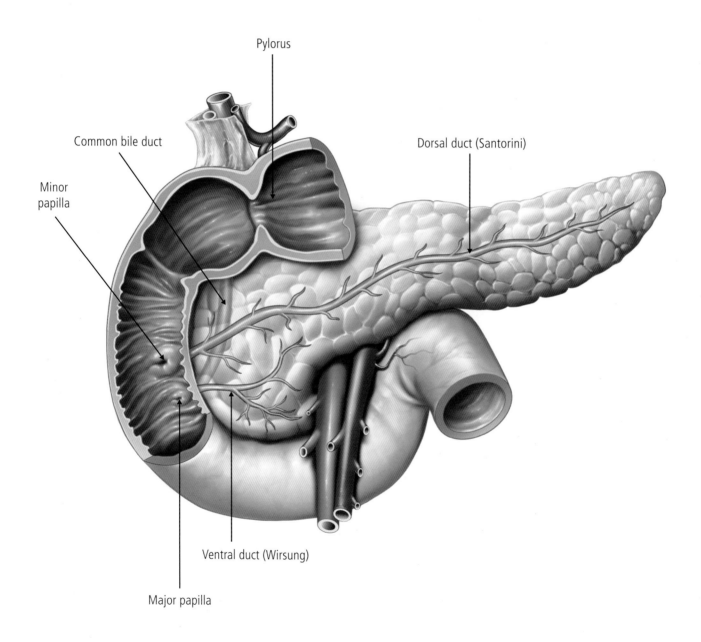

Pylorus

Common bile duct

Dorsal duct (Santorini)

Minor
papilla

Ventral duct (Wirsung)

Major papilla

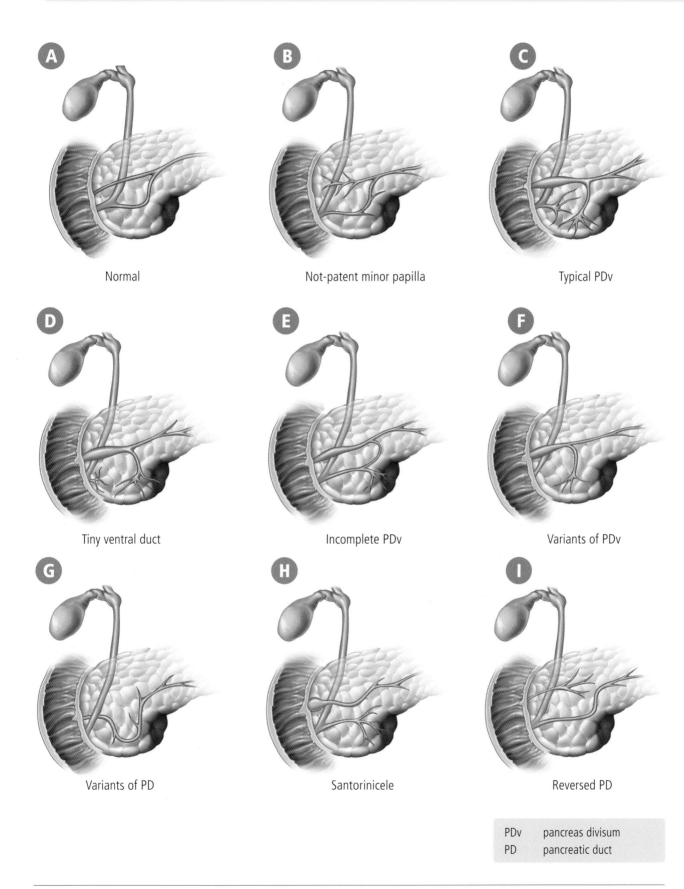

A — Normal

B — Not-patent minor papilla

C — Typical PDv

D — Tiny ventral duct

E — Incomplete PDv

F — Variants of PDv

G — Variants of PD

H — Santorinicele

I — Reversed PD

PDv	pancreas divisum
PD	pancreatic duct

Normal and variant anatomy of pancreatic duct

02 Annular pancreas

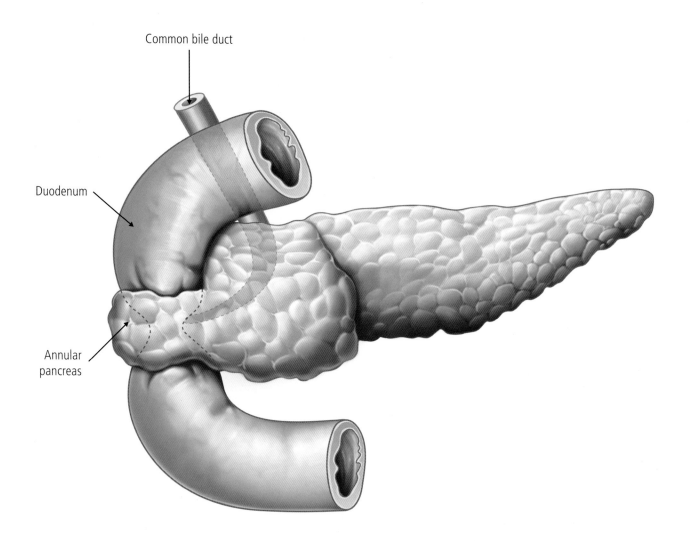

Common bile duct

Duodenum

Annular
pancreas

Annular pancreas with duodenal obstruction

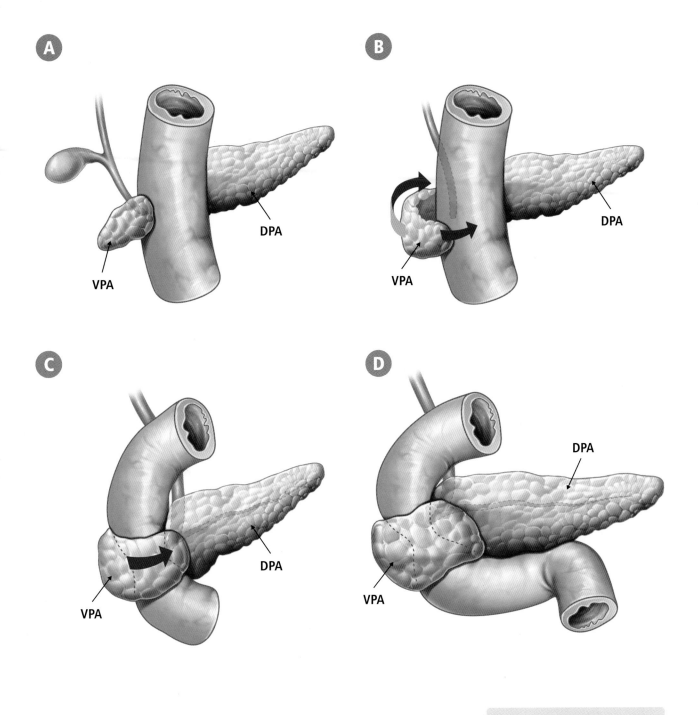

VPA   ventral pancreatic anlage
DPA   dorsal pancreatic anlage

Development of annular pancreas

03 Chronic pancreatitis

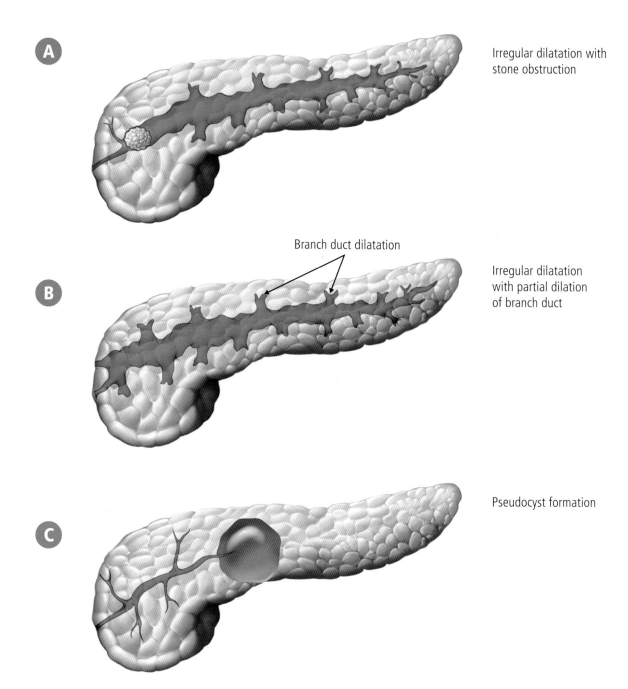

A — Irregular dilatation with stone obstruction

Branch duct dilatation

B — Irregular dilatation with partial dilation of branch duct

C — Pseudocyst formation

Pancreatographic features of chronic pancreatitis

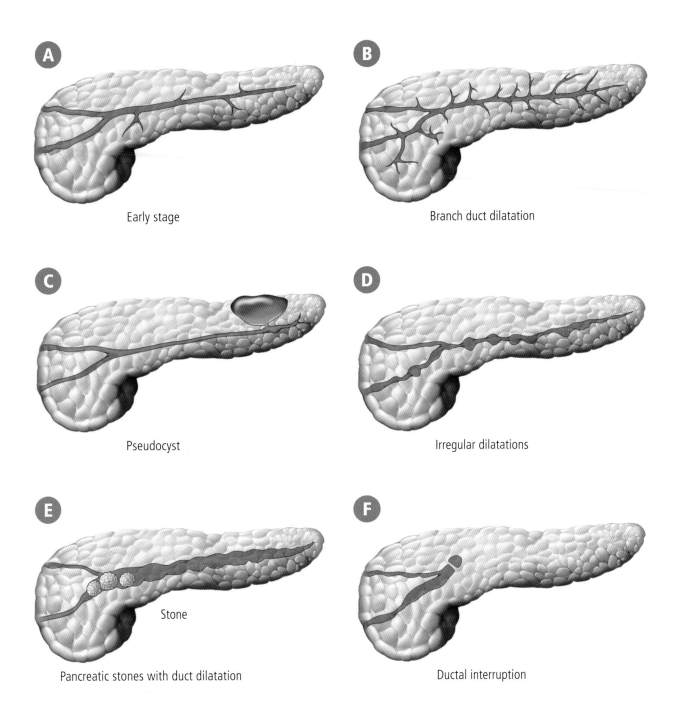

A — Early stage

B — Branch duct dilatation

C — Pseudocyst

D — Irregular dilatations

E — Pancreatic stones with duct dilatation / Stone

F — Ductal interruption

Pancreatographic features of chronic pancreatitis

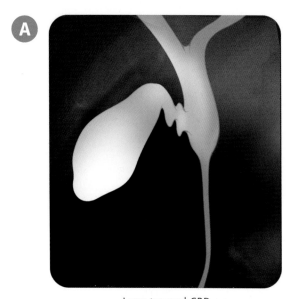

Long tapered CBD

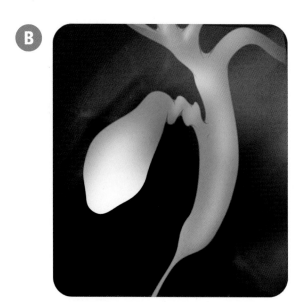

Smooth stricture of distal CBD

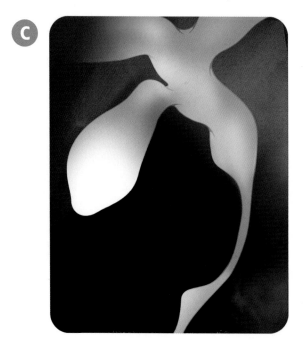

Extrinsic compression

CBD   common bile duct

Cholangiographic features of chronic pancreatitis

04 Pancreas cystic lesion

Locularity

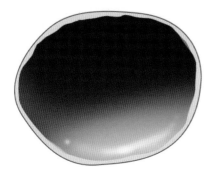

Unilocular with
smooth contour

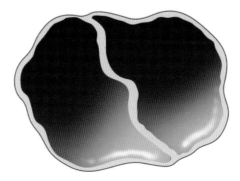

Bilocular with lobulating
contour and thick septum

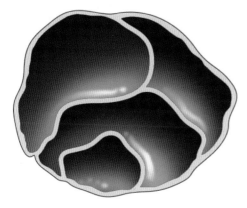

Oligolocular

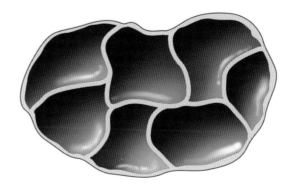

Multilocular

Morphology of panreas cystic lesions (1)

Size of cysts

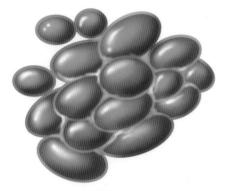

Multiple
microcysts

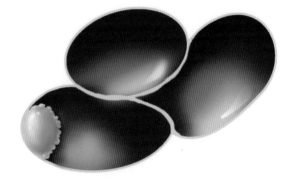

Macrocysts with
mural nodule

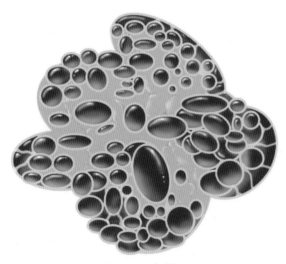

Honeycomb-like
appearance

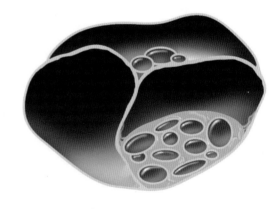

Mixed micro-and
macrocysts

Morphology of panreas cystic lesions (2)

Communication with pancreatic duct

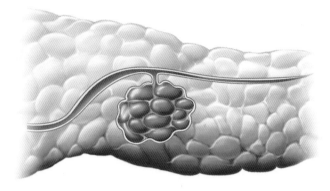

Branch-duct IPMN;
grape-like cluster with
communication

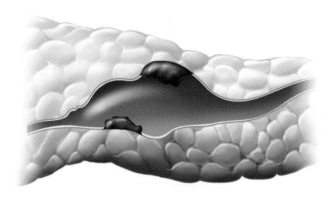

Main-duct IPMN:
Saccular dilation of
main pancreatic duct with mass

IPMN   intraductal papillary mucinous neoplasm

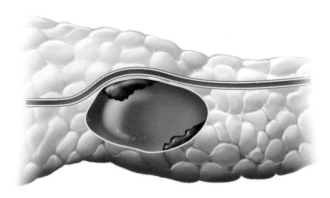

Mucinous cystadenocarcinoma
without communication

Morphology of panreas cystic lesions (3)

05 Pancreatic cancer

Obstructive type

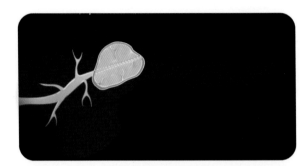

Stenotic type

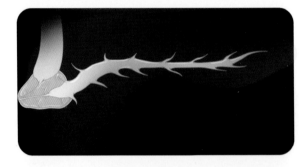

Diffuse narrowing type

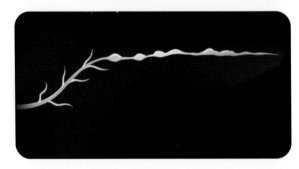

Abnormal branching type

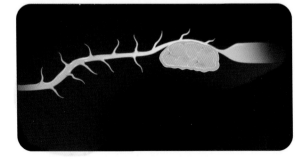

Pancreatographic findings of pancreatic cancer

06 Autoimmune pancreatitis

Diffuse stricture

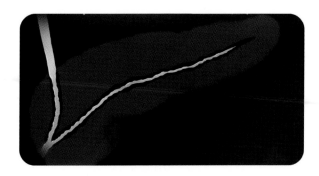

Focal stricture

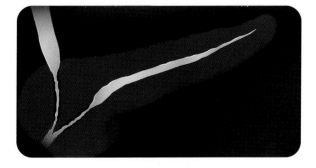

Multifocal strictures

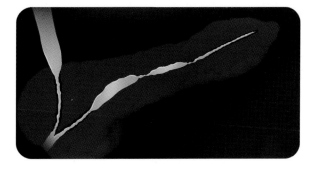

Pancreatographic findings of autoimmune pancreatitis

Techniques of ERCP

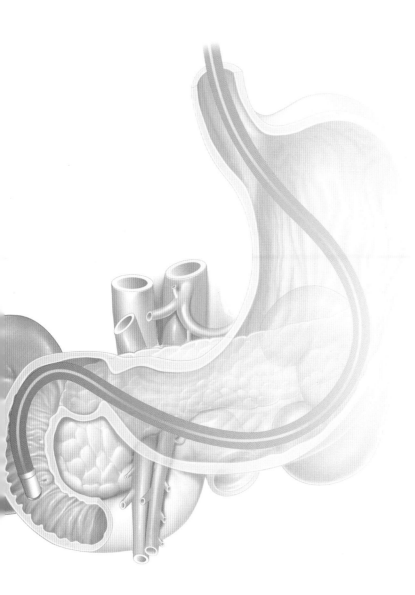

01 Intubation of duodenoscope

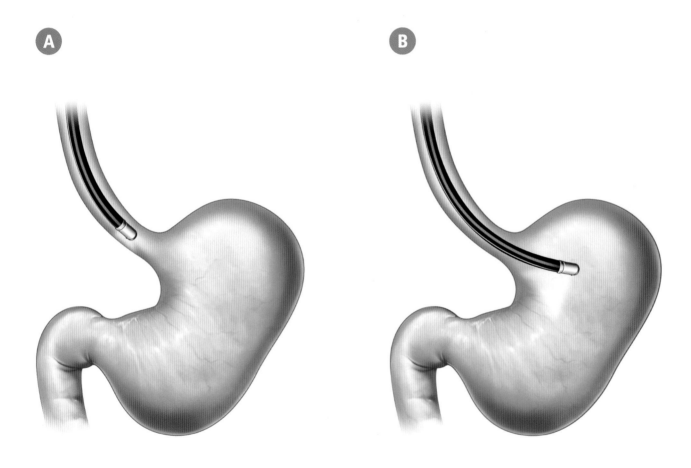

A) Gentle downward tip angulation allows examination of the distal esophagus.

B) The stomach is slightly inflated to allow an adequate view of the lumen. The endoscope is slowly advanced with tip angled downwards looking at the greater curvature and distal stomach.

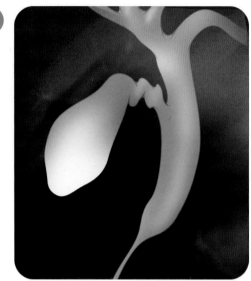

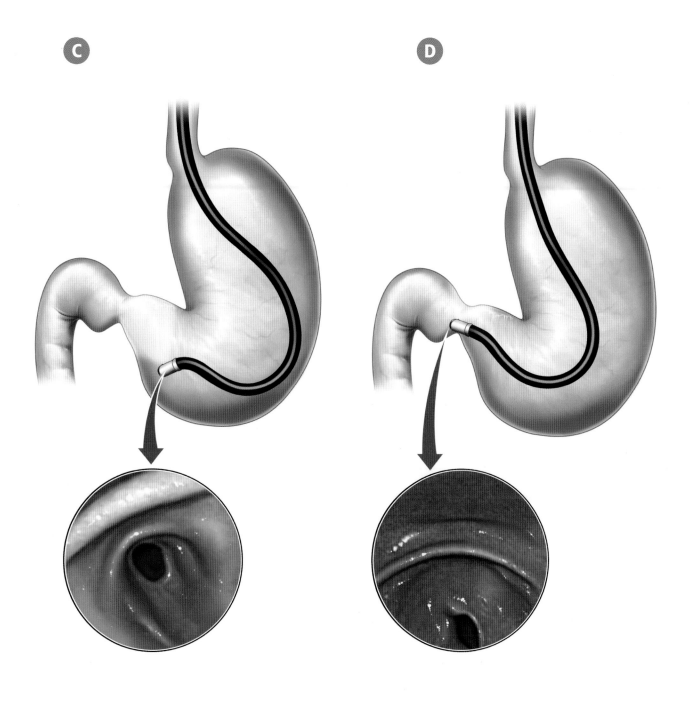

C) Reach the pyloric ring by advancing the scope while looking at the lesser curvature.

D) To pass through the pyloric ring, advance the scope with up angle while positioning pyloric ring at 6 o'clock.

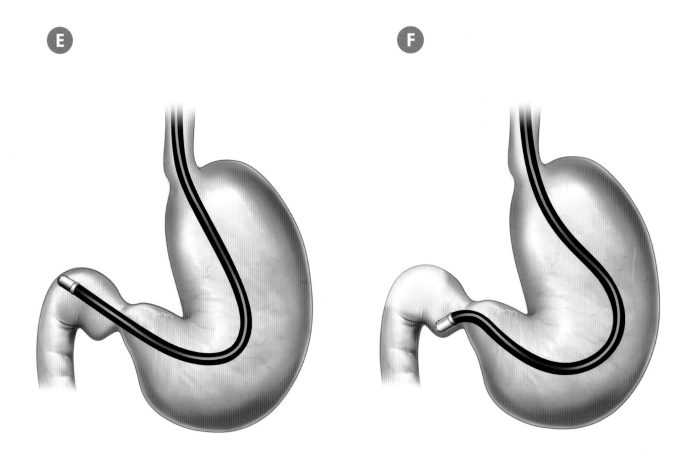

E) When the scope passes through the pyloric ring, the tip of the scope comes in contact with duodenal wall.

F) Use down angle and retract the scope to find the duodenal lumen.

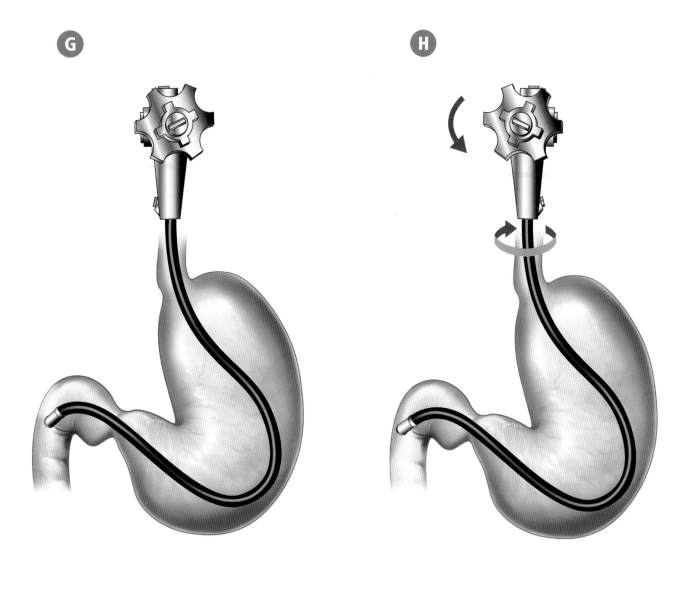

G) Pass the superior duodenal angle by advancing the scope with up angle.

H) Rotating the scope in clockwise direction with up and right angle allows visualization of the descending duodenum.

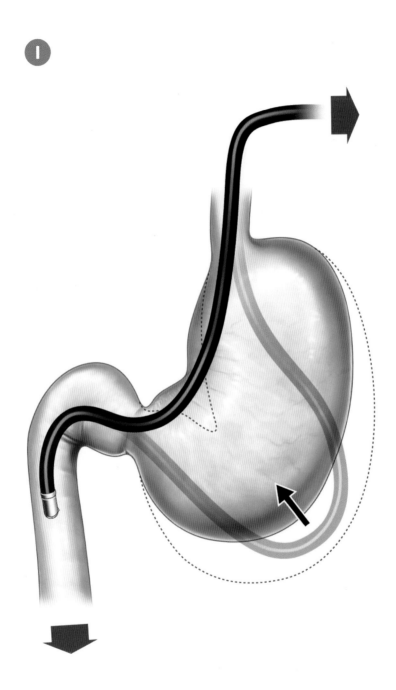

I) To advance the scope into the 2nd portion of duodenum, gently withdraw it while maintaining visualization of duodenal lumen.

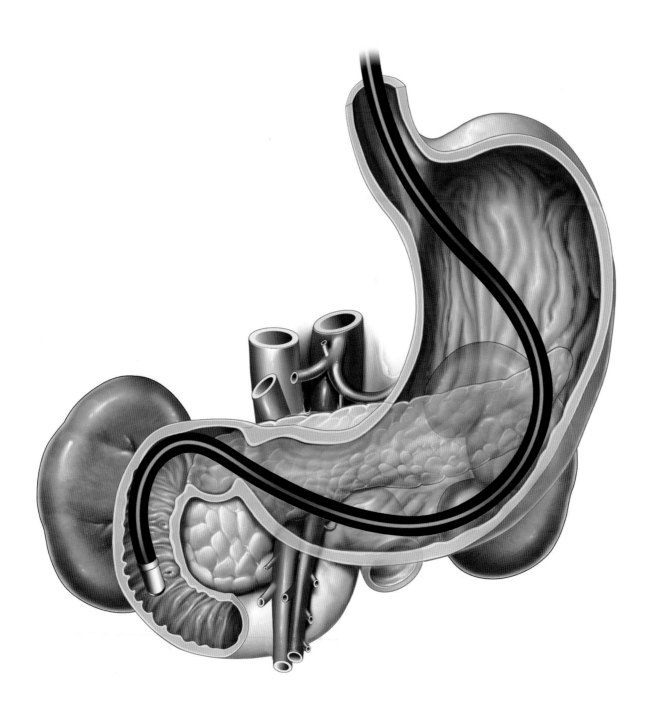

Long loop position

02 Cannulation

❶ Conventional method

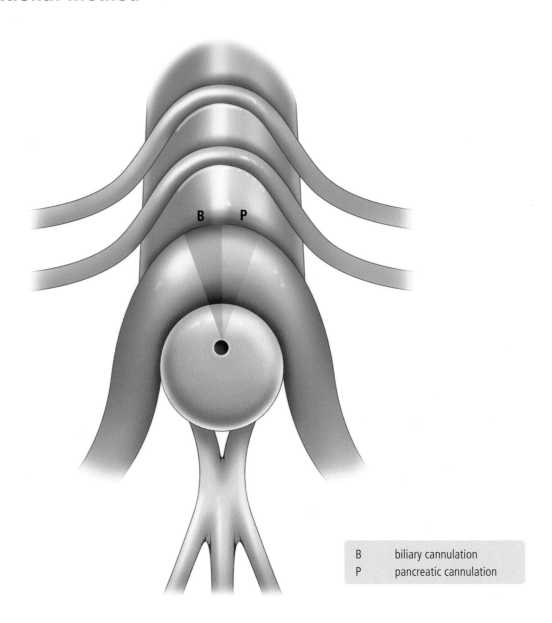

B P

| B | biliary cannulation |
| P | pancreatic cannulation |

Axes of biliary and pancreatic duct

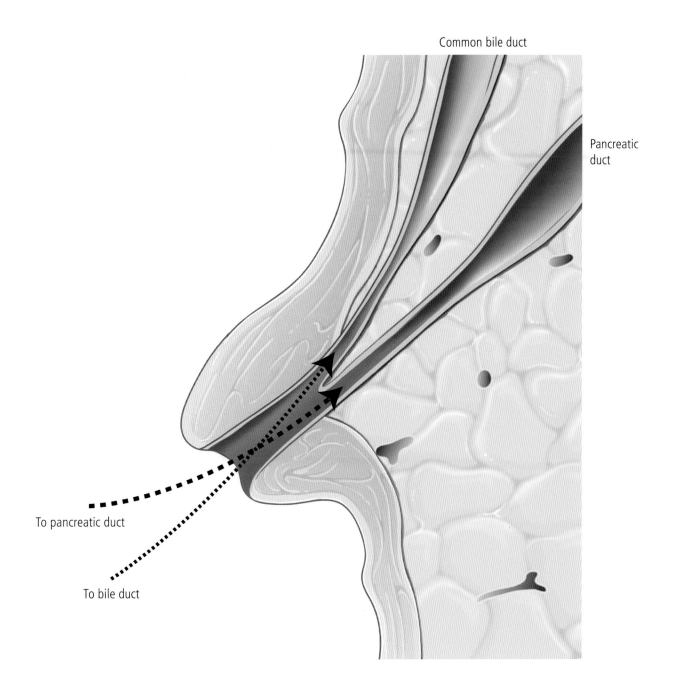

Common bile duct

Pancreatic
duct

To pancreatic duct

To bile duct

Vertical axes of deep cannulation

Common bile duct

Pancreatic duct

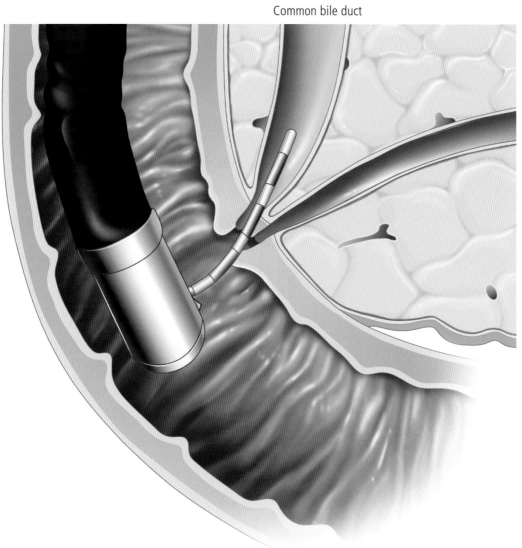

Bile duct cannulation

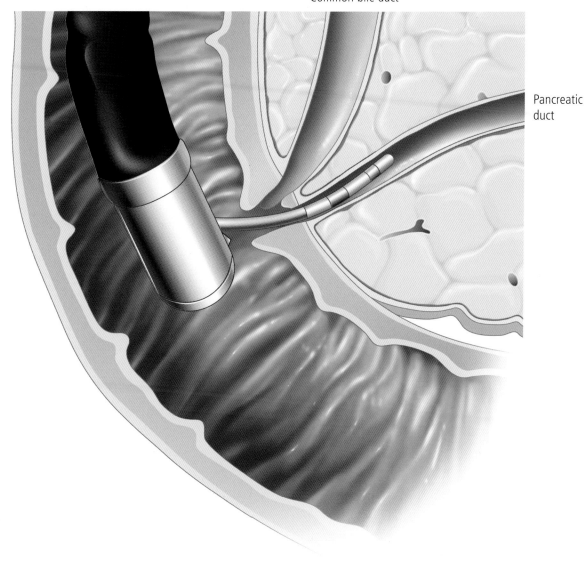

Common bile duct

Pancreatic
duct

Pancreatic duct cannulation

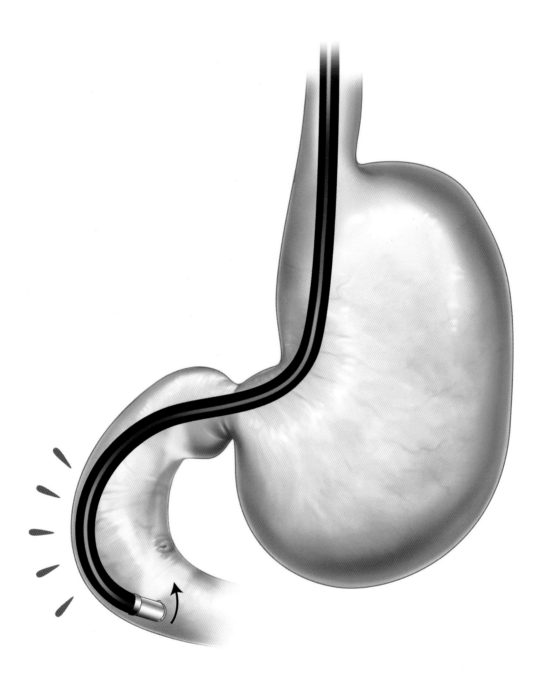

With the scope in the straight position, angle the tip up.

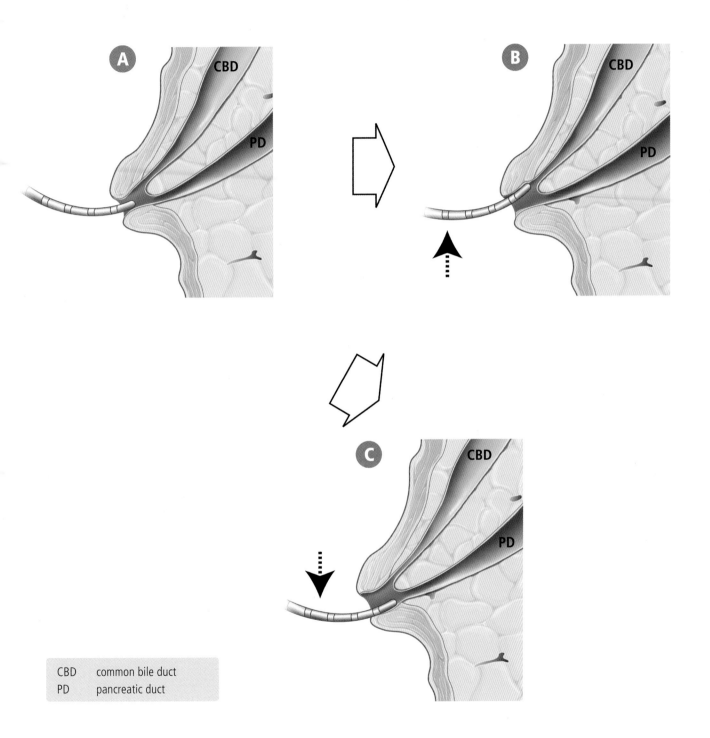

CBD   common bile duct
PD   pancreatic duct

A) From the central catheter position, B) Lift up for the bile duct, C) Drop down for the pancreatic duct

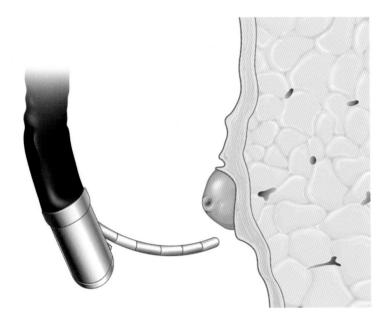

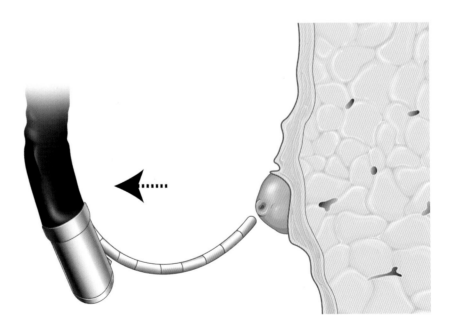

Biliary access may be facilitated by approaching the major papilla using the natural curve of the cannula.

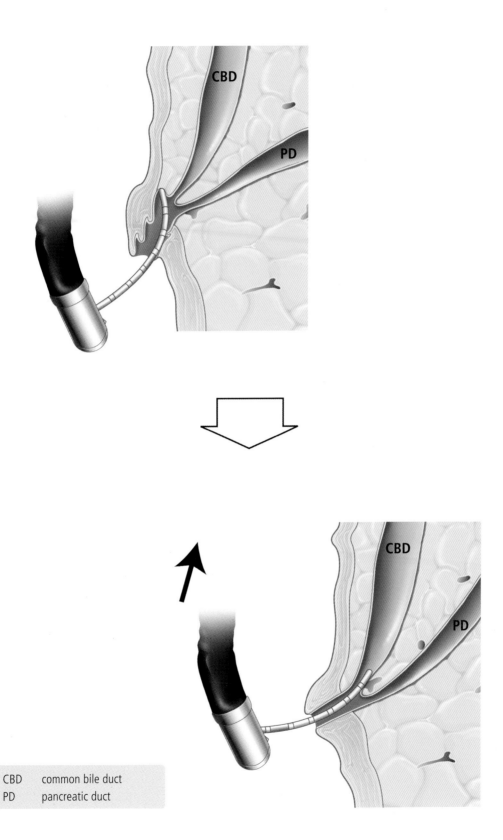

| CBD | common bile duct |
| PD | pancreatic duct |

Pull the scope back to set the axis for proper biliary cannulation.

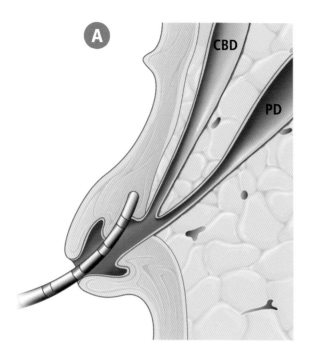

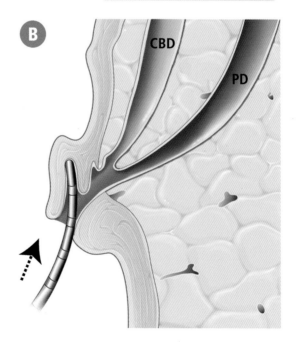

CBD	common bile duct
PD	pancreatic duct

A) Wrong axis of deep cannulation

B) Too much emphasis on pushing up from below is counterproductive.

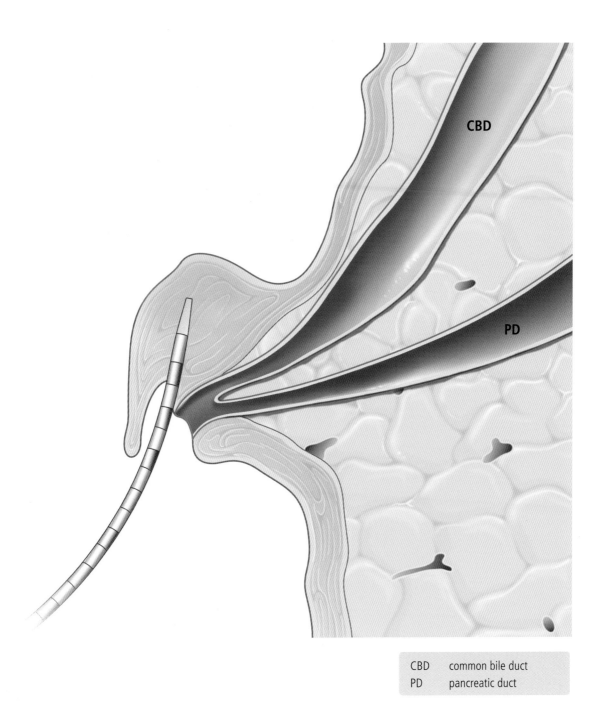

| CBD | common bile duct |
| PD | pancreatic duct |

Erroneous submucosal injection due to a sharp taper-tipped cannula

❷ Cannulation using papillotome

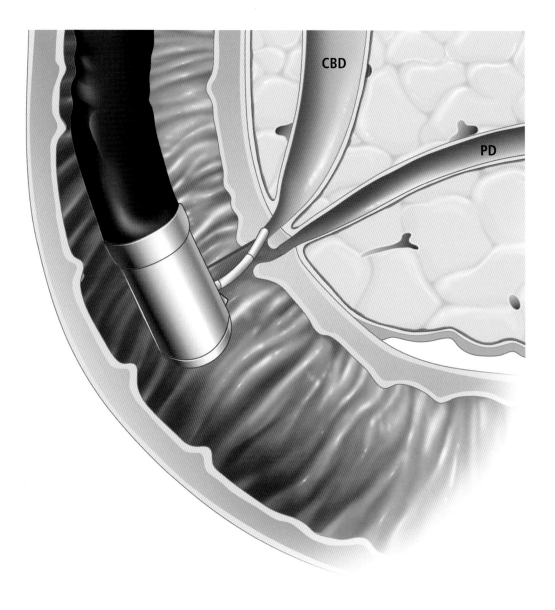

| CBD | common bile duct |
| PD | pancreatic duct |

Biliary cannulation using papillotome

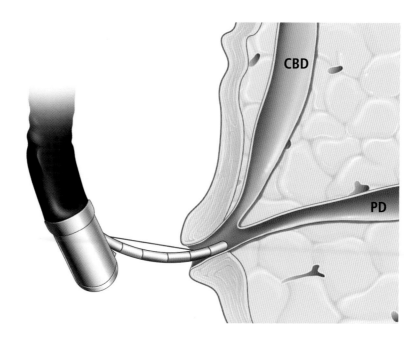

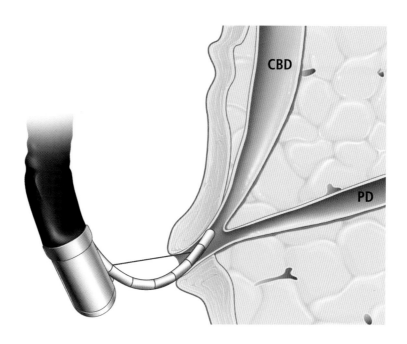

Bowing papillotome helps to achieve correct axis.

❸ Guidewire technique

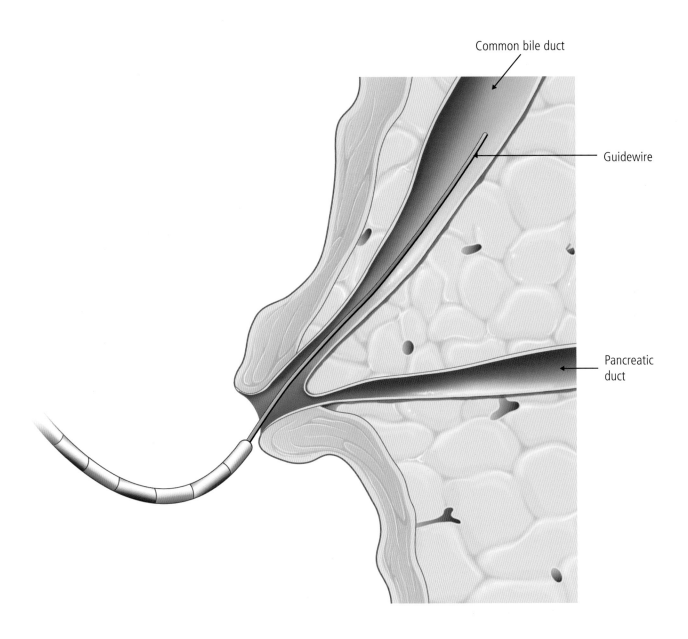

Common bile duct

Guidewire

Pancreatic duct

Guidewire-assisted cannulation

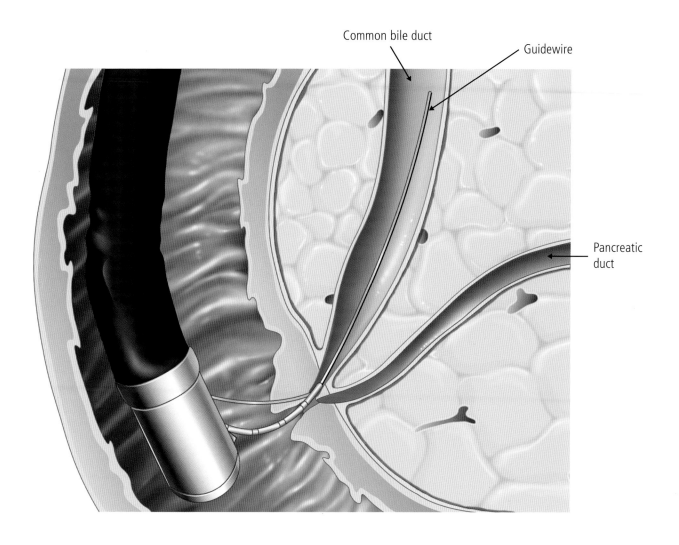

Common bile duct

Guidewire

Pancreatic
duct

Papillotome and guidewire-assisted biliary cannulation

❹ Wire-in-pancreatic duct technique

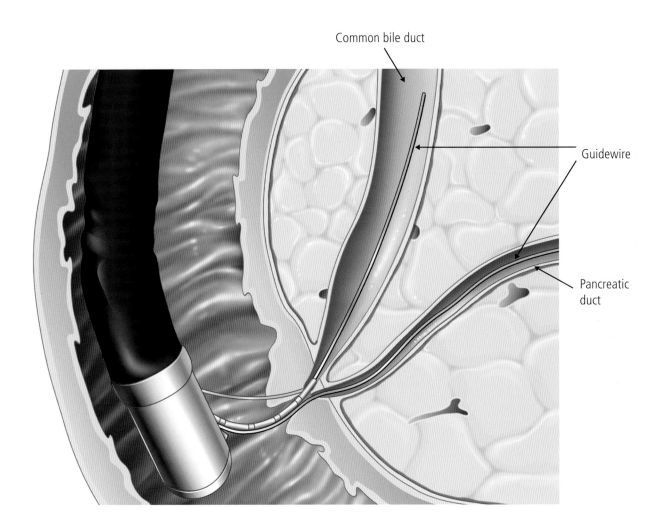

Common bile duct

Guidewire

Pancreatic duct

Double guidewire technique for biliary cannulation (papillotome-assisted)

❺ Stent-in-pancreatic duct technique

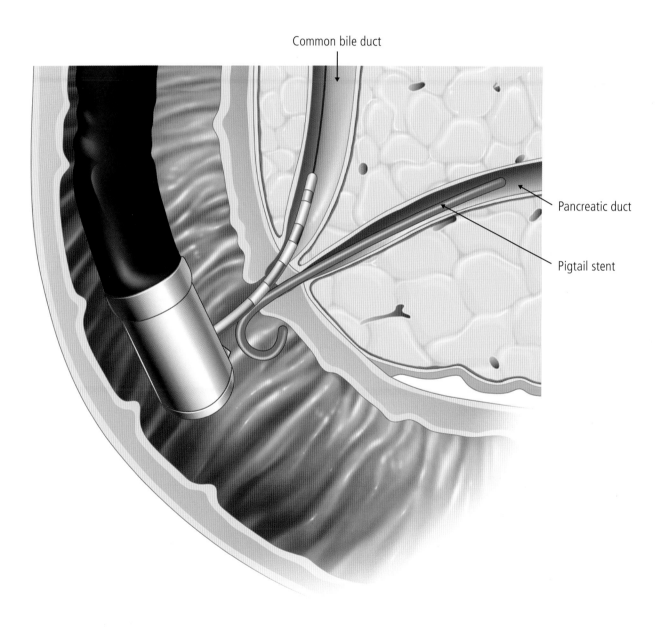

Common bile duct

Pancreatic duct

Pigtail stent

03 / Altered anatomy

❶ Subtotal gastrectomy

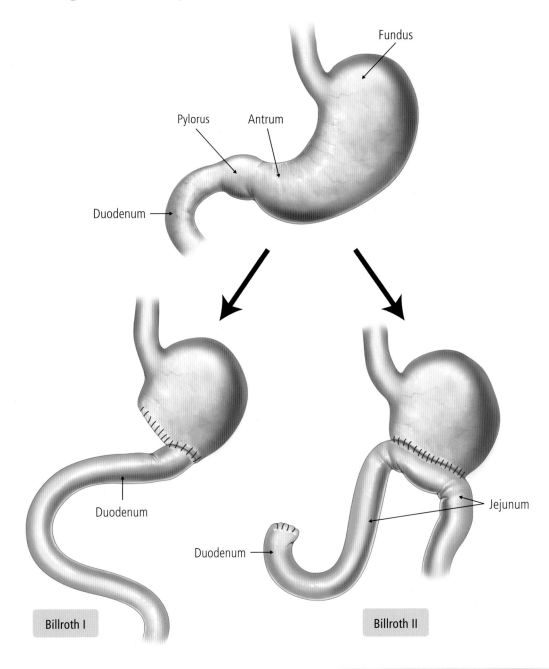

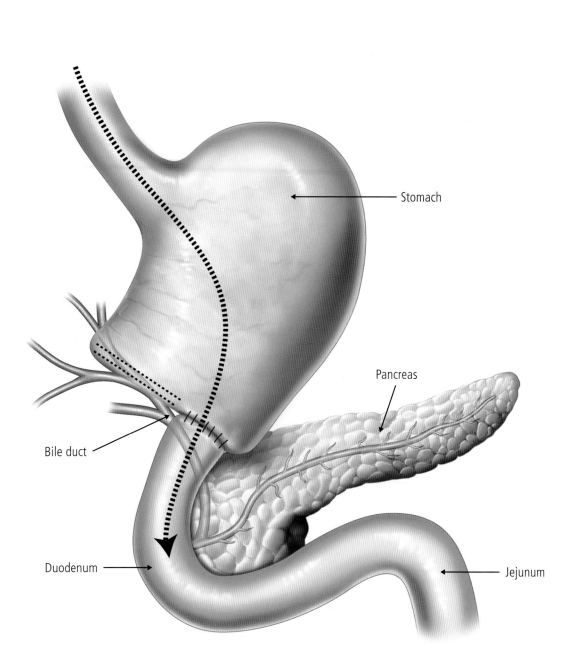

Stomach

Pancreas

Bile duct

Duodenum

Jejunum

Billroth I gastrectomy

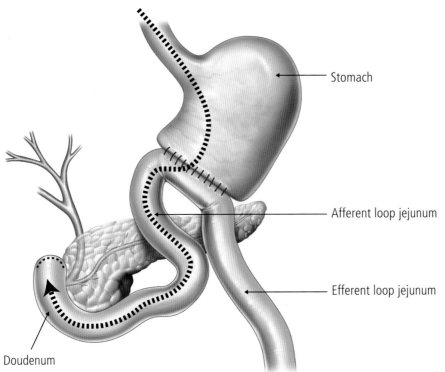

Stomach

Afferent loop jejunum

Efferent loop jejunum

Doudenum

Antiperistaltic anastomosis

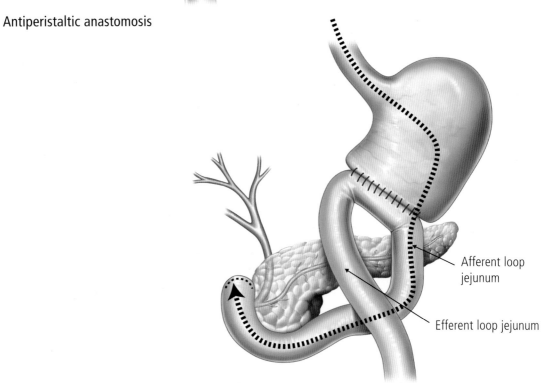

Afferent loop jejunum

Efferent loop jejunum

Isoperistaltic anastomosis

Billroth II gastrectomy

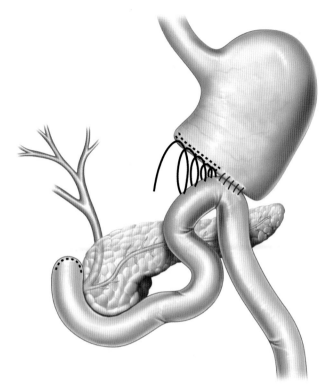

End-to-side gastrojejunostomy

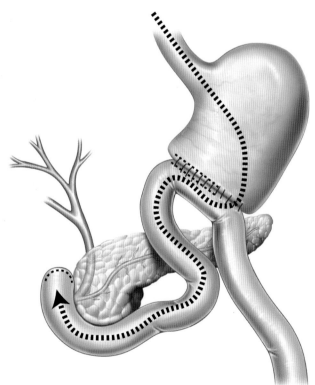

Suture the jejunum onto the lesser
curvature side of the stomach

Modification of Billoth II gastrectomy

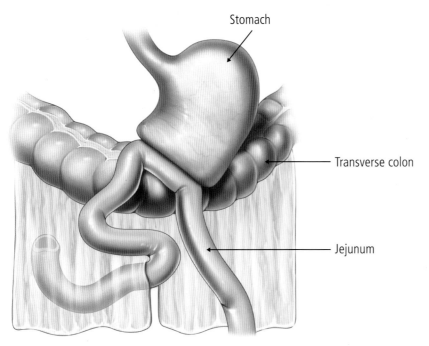

Stomach

Transverse colon

Jejunum

Antecolic construction

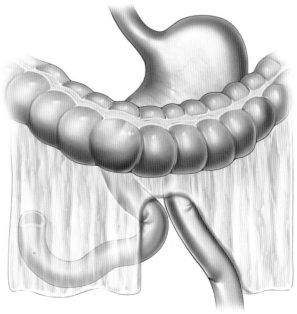

Retrocolic construction

Billroth II gastrectomy

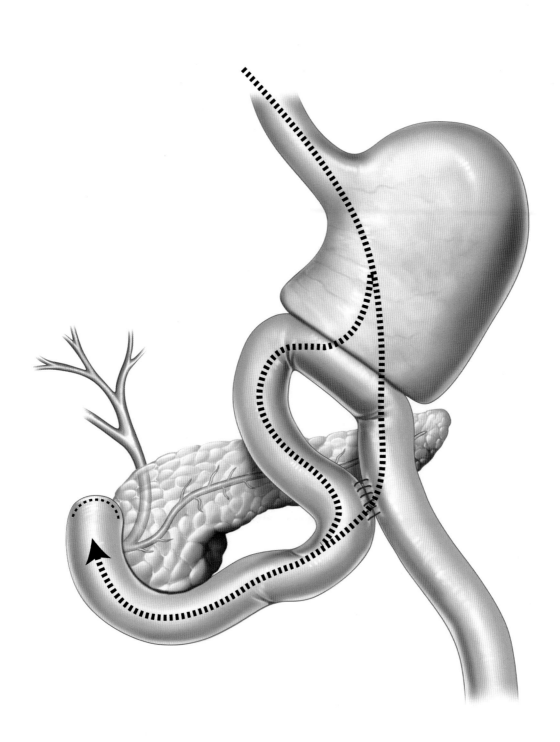

Braun modification of Billroth II gastrectomy

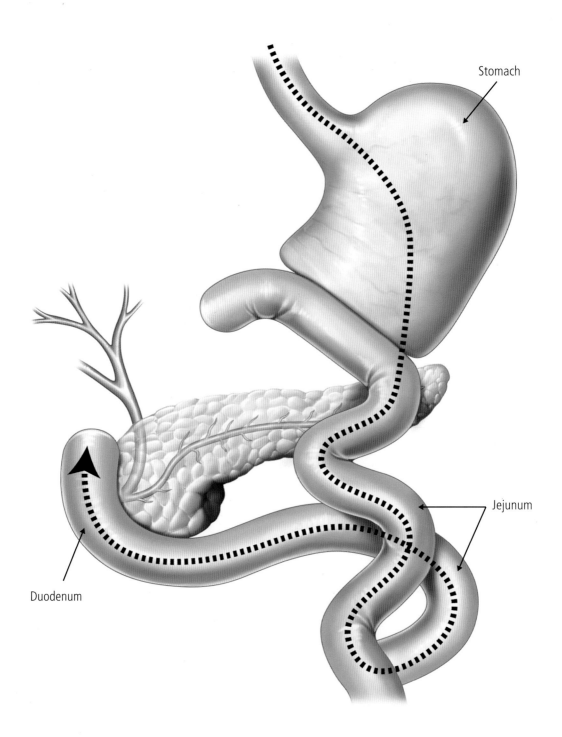

Stomach

Jejunum

Duodenum

Roux-en-Y gastrojejunostomy

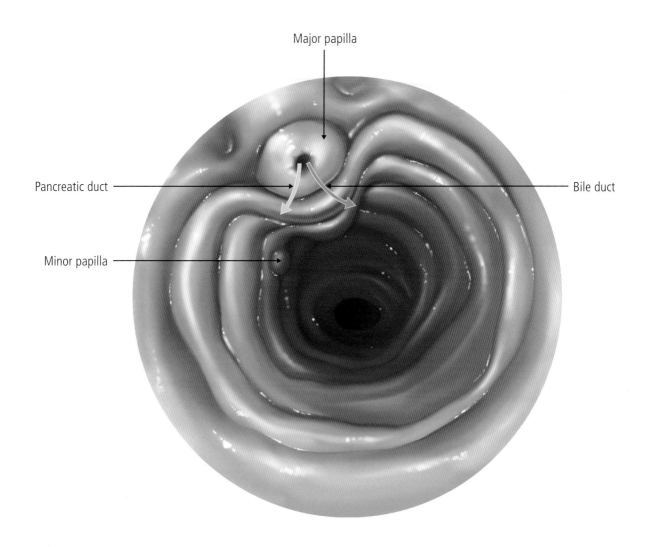

Major papilla

Pancreatic duct

Bile duct

Minor papilla

B-II gastrectomy results in inverted orientation of major papilla.

Minor papilla is located distal to major papilla. Direction of the bile duct (green arrow) and pancreatic duct (yellow arrow)

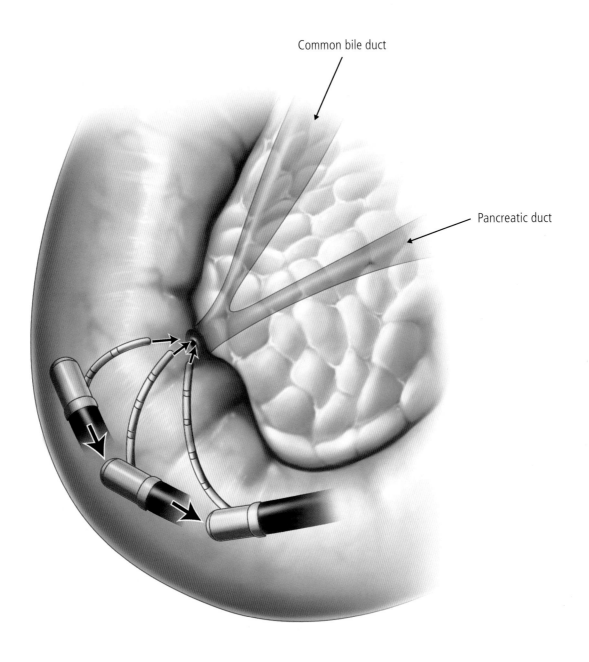

Common bile duct

Pancreatic duct

Withdrawing the scope produces a better cannulation axis but a more distant approach.

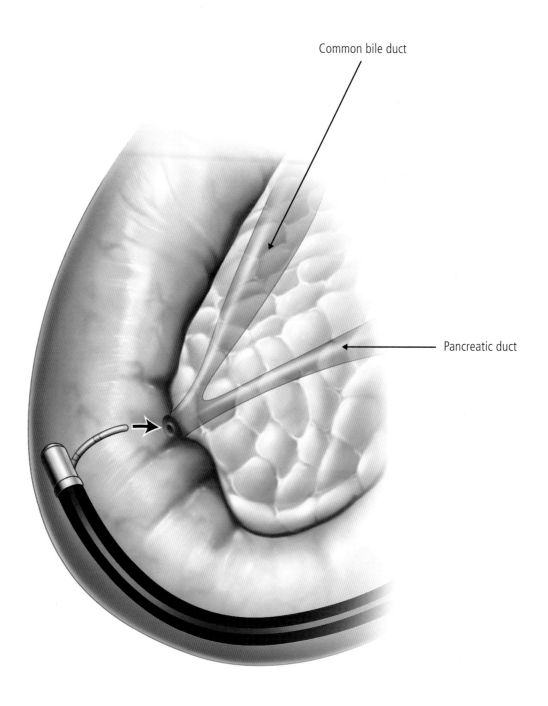

Common bile duct

Pancreatic duct

The natural curve of the cannula is unhelpful.

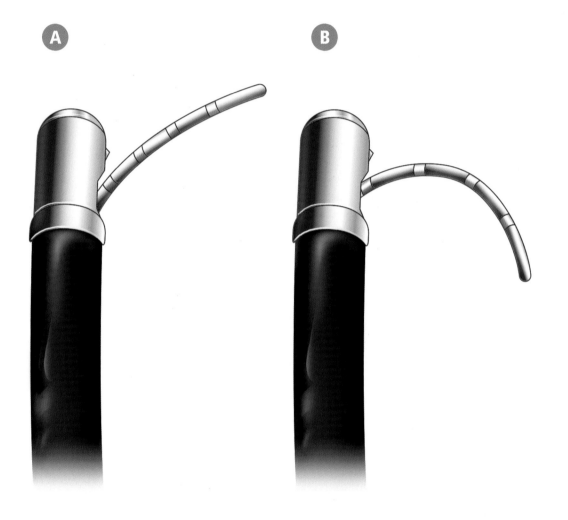

A new cannula tends to curl less then an old one.

A) New, B) Used

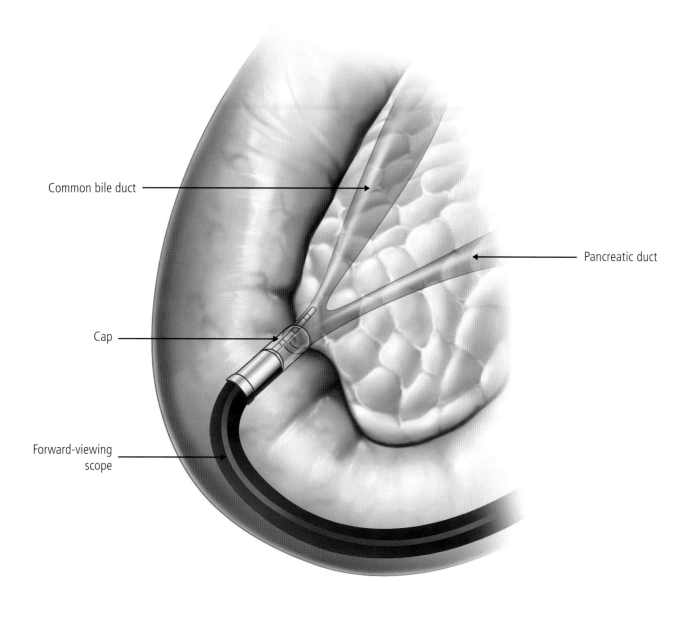

Common bile duct

Pancreatic duct

Cap

Forward-viewing
scope

Cap-assisted technique with forward-viewing scope for Billroth II anastomosis

❷ Total gastrectomy

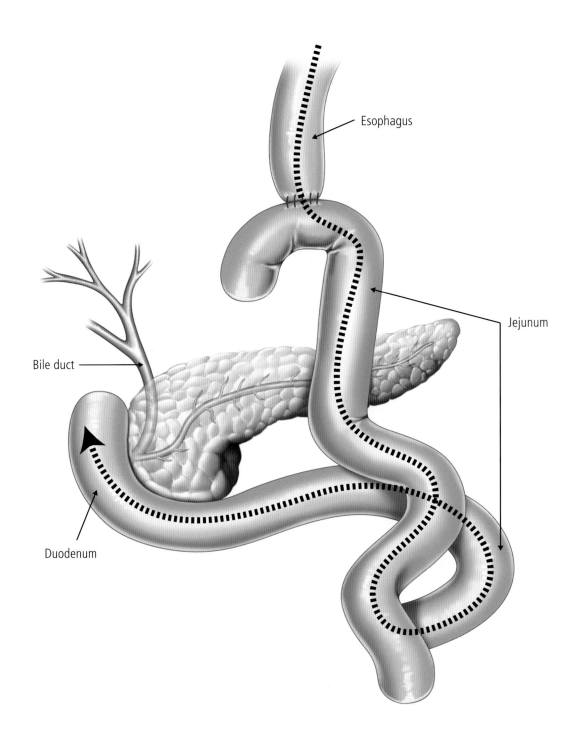

Esophagus

Jejunum

Bile duct

Duodenum

Total gastrectomy with Roux-en-Y esophagojejunostomy

❸ Pancreaticoduodenectomy

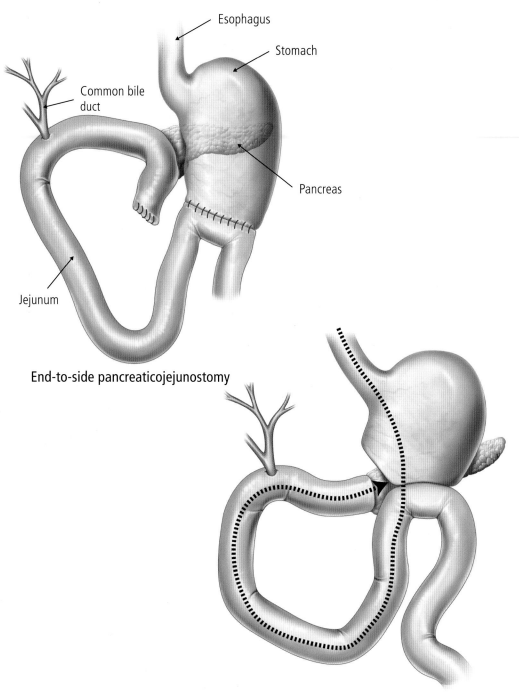

Esophagus

Stomach

Common bile
duct

Pancreas

Jejunum

End-to-side pancreaticojejunostomy

End-to-end pancreaticojejunostomy

Classic Whipple operation

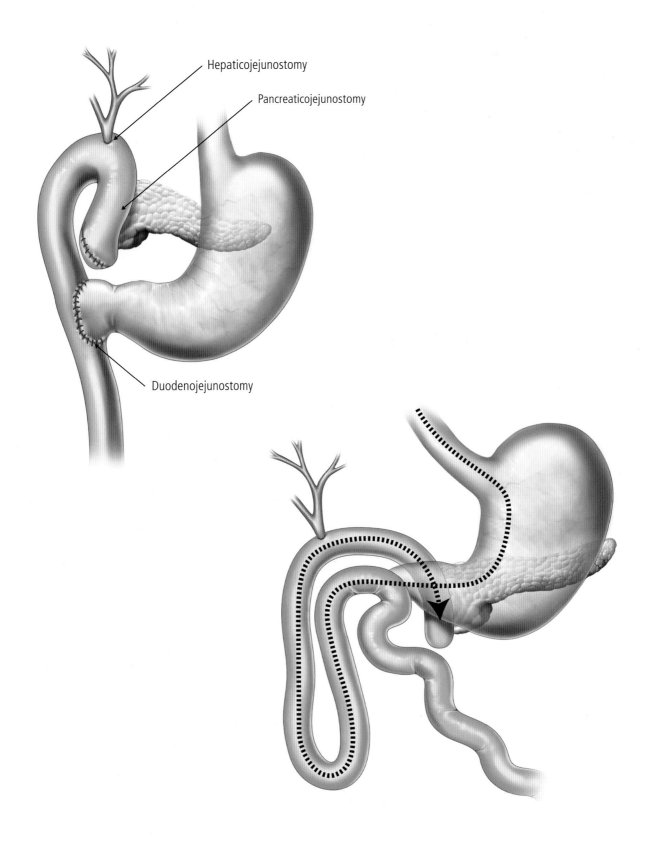

Hepaticojejunostomy

Pancreaticojejunostomy

Duodenojejunostomy

Pylorus-preserving pancreaticoduodenectomy (PPPD)

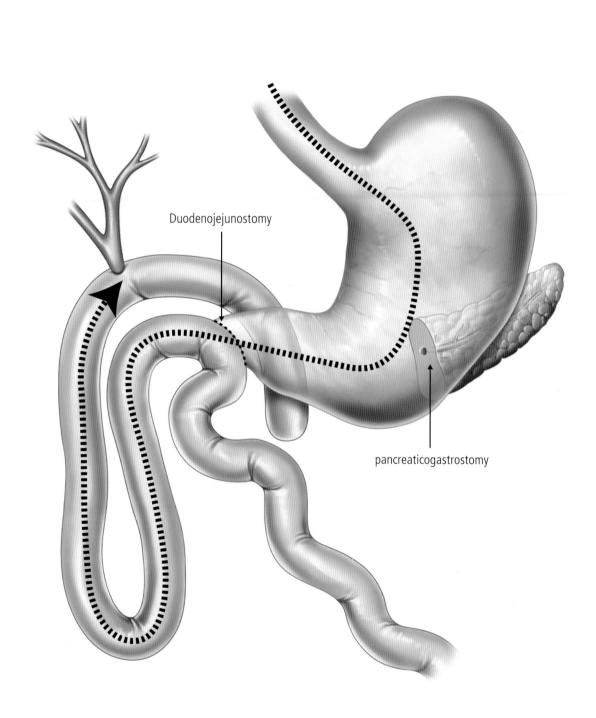

Duodenojejunostomy

pancreaticogastrostomy

PPPD with pancreaticogastrostomy

❹ Bariatric surgery

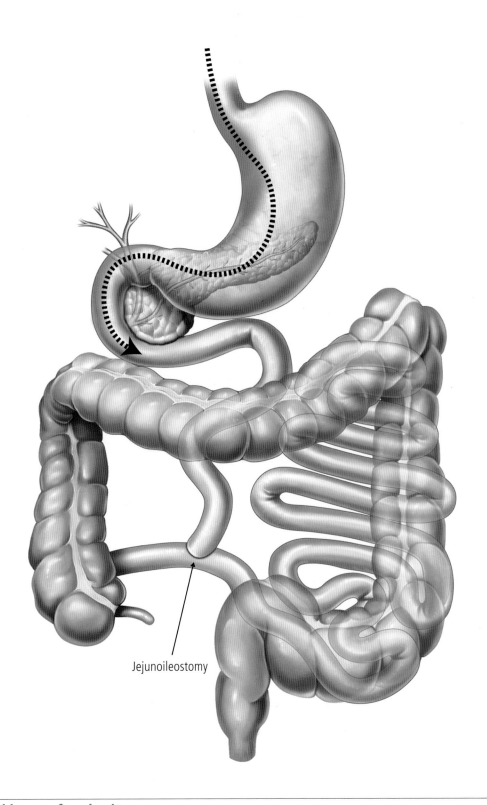

Jejunoileostomy

Jejunoileal bypass for obesity

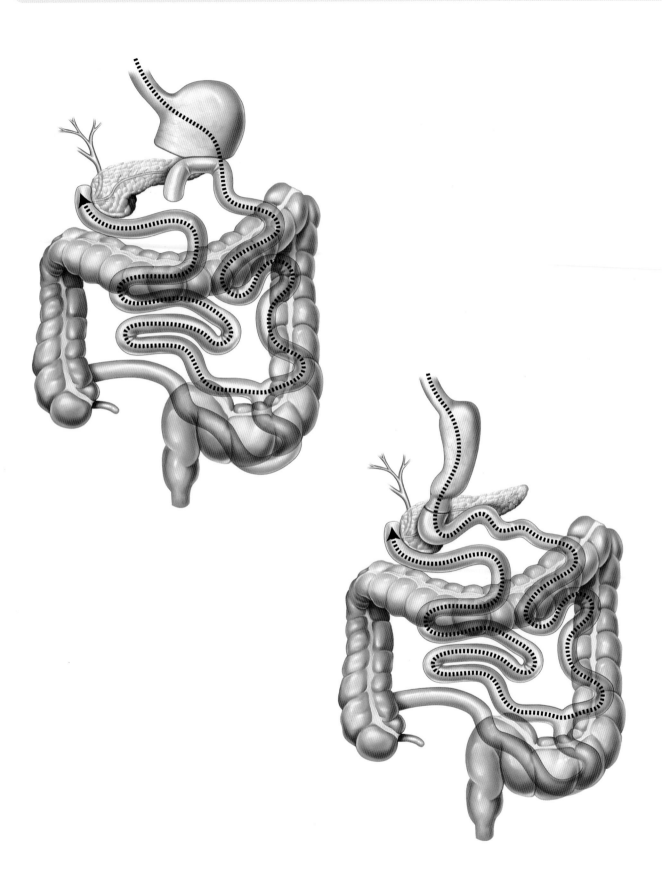

Biliopancreatic diversion for obesity

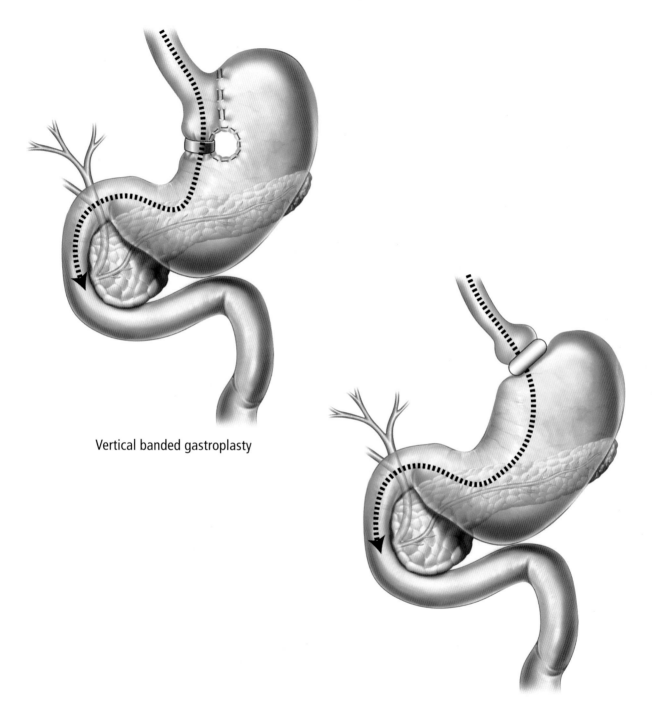

Vertical banded gastroplasty

Laparoscopic gastric banding

Restrictive surgery for obesity

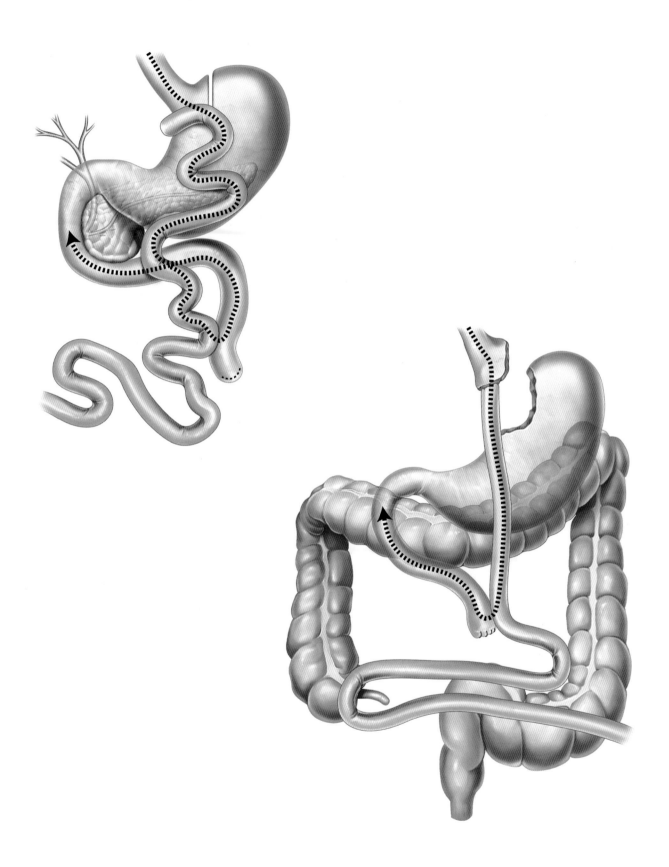

Gastric bypass for obesity

❺ Other operations

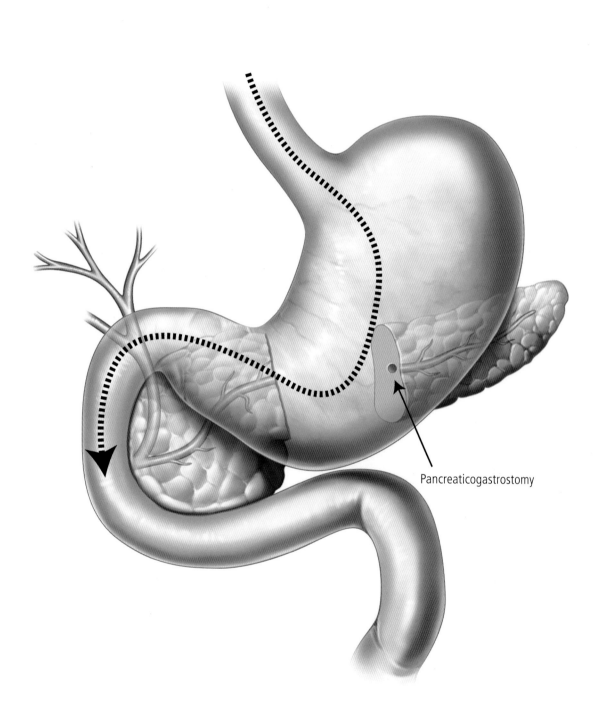

Pancreaticogastrostomy

Pancreaticogastrostomy

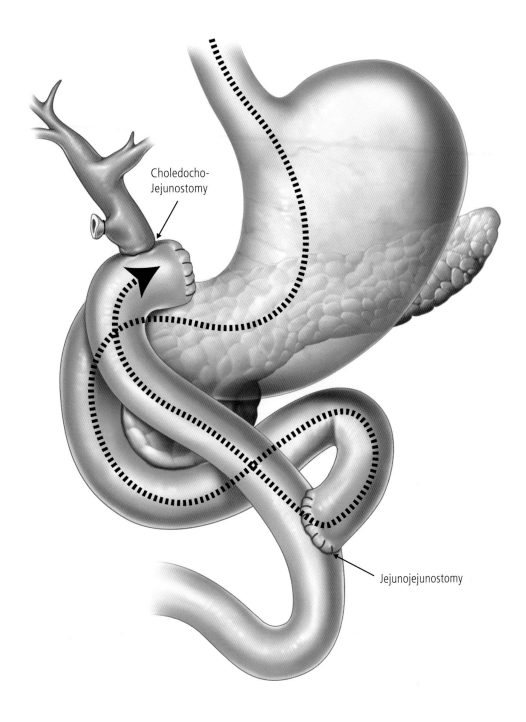

Choledocho-
Jejunostomy

Jejunojejunostomy

Choledochojejunostomy

❻ Periampullary diverticulum

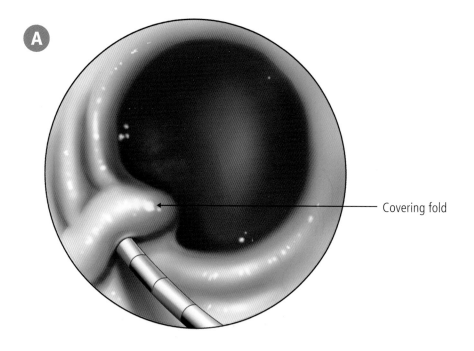

Covering fold

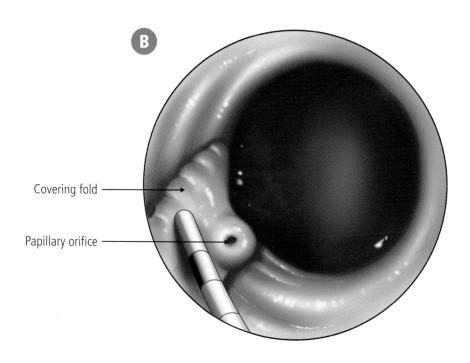

Covering fold

Papillary orifice

A) Push with the catheter or papillotome to evert the papilla from diverticulum.
B) Further pressure laterally brings the orifice into view.

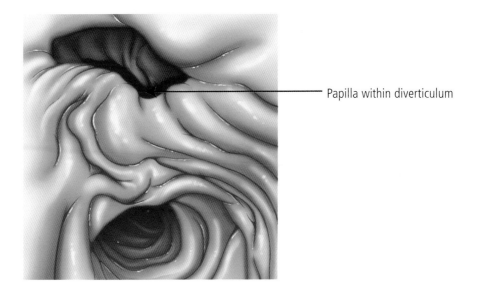

Papilla within diverticulum

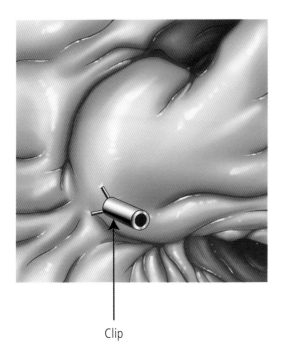

Clip

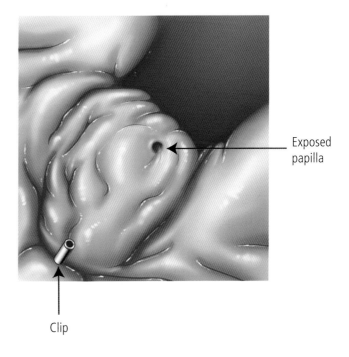

Exposed papilla

Clip

Clip-assisted biliary cannulation for major papilla within a duodenal diverticulum

04 Precut

❶ Conventional method

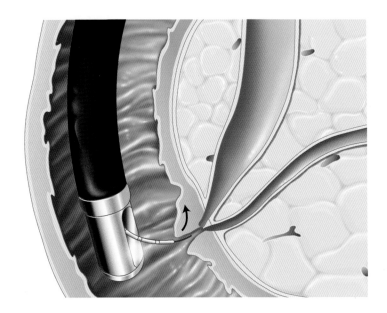

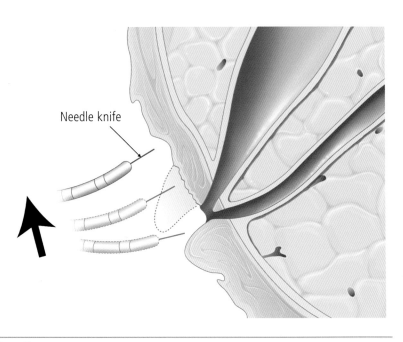

Needle knife

Incision from the orifice in upward direction

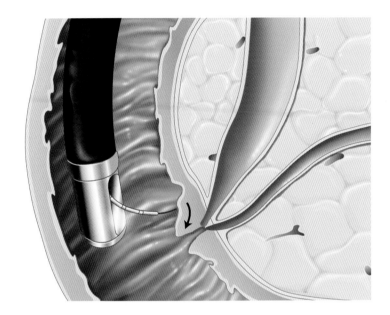

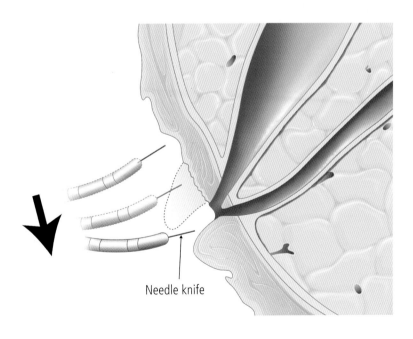

Needle knife

Incision from papillary roof in downward direction

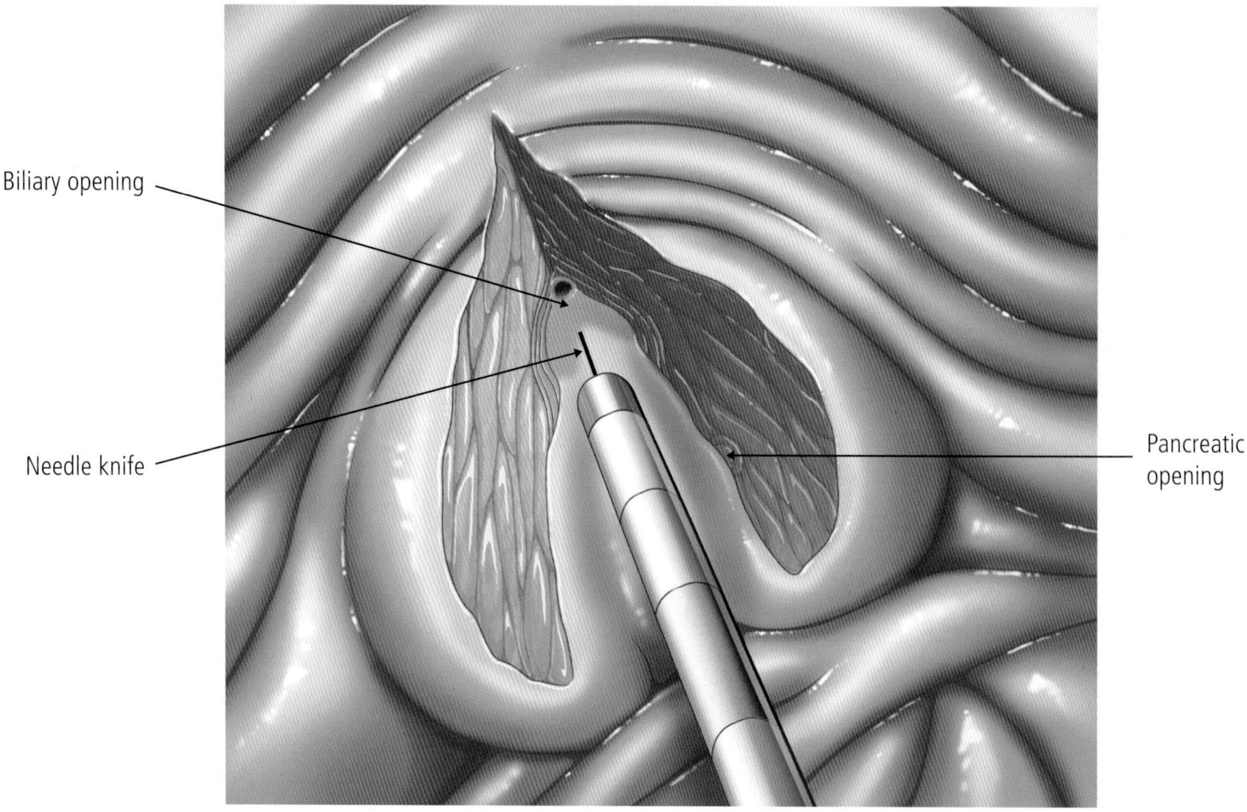

Biliary opening

Needle knife

Pancreatic opening

Concept of sphincterotomy using needle knife

Incision forms inverted "V" shape

Pancreatic opening at right inferior and biliary opening at left superior aspect

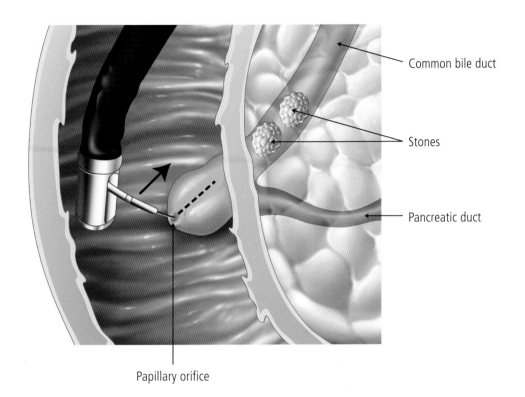

Common bile duct

Stones

Pancreatic duct

Papillary orifice

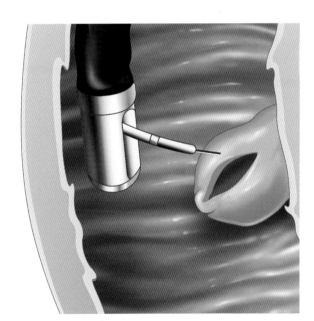

Coronal section image of precut papillotomy using needle knife

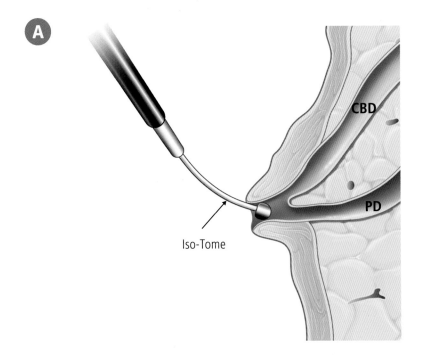

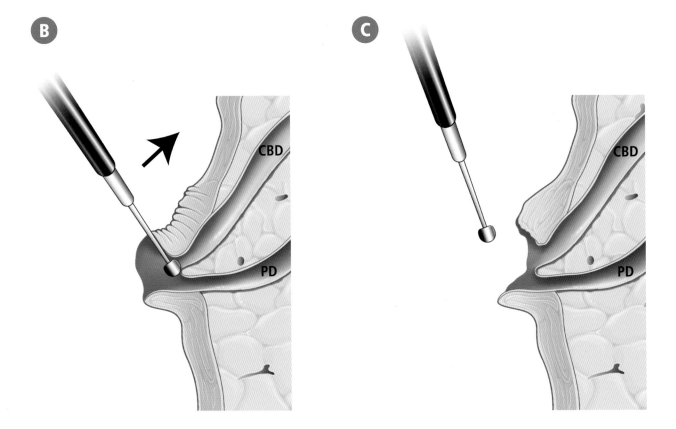

CBD   common bile duct
PD   pancreatic duct

Precut papillotomy with Iso-Tome®

A) Placing in the orifice of the ampulla of Vater, B) Pushing toward the papillary roof, C) After precutting

❷ Infundibulotomy

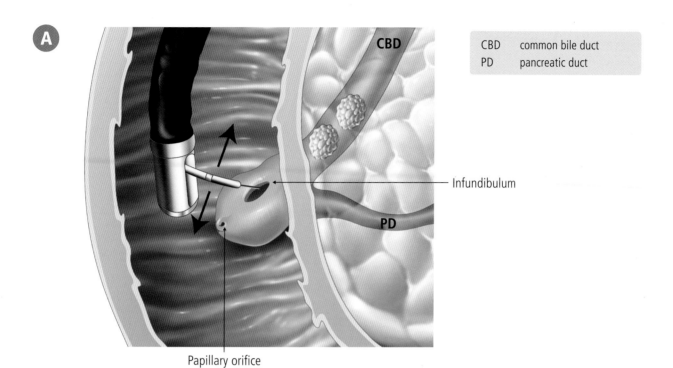

| CBD | common bile duct |
| PD | pancreatic duct |

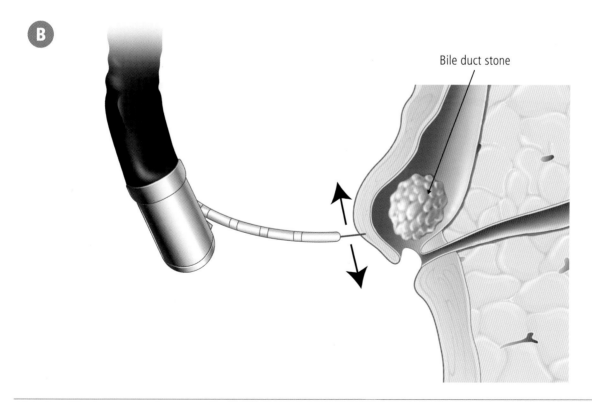

A) Infundibulotomy using needle knife
B) Infundibulotomy can be performed in either oral or caudal direction.

❸ Transpancreatic precut sphincterotomy (Transpancreatic papillary septotomy)

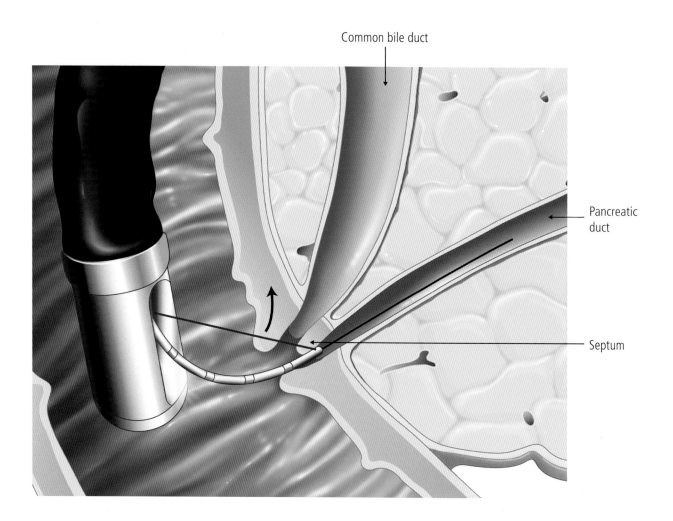

Common bile duct

Pancreatic duct

Septum

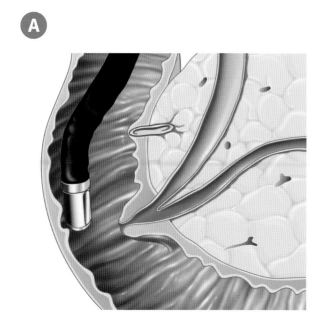

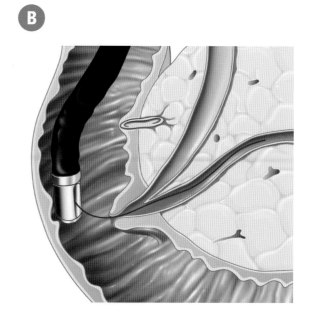

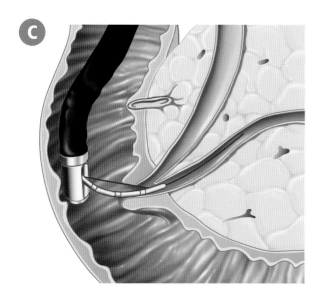

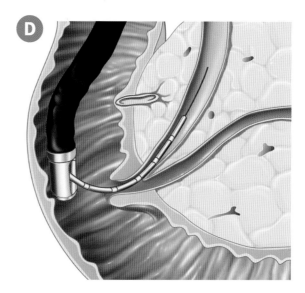

Transpancreatic precut sphincterotomy for selective cannulation of bile duct

❹ Precut along the pancreatic duct stent

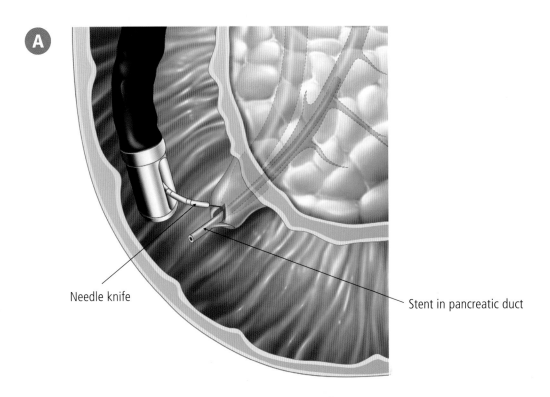

A

Needle knife

Stent in pancreatic duct

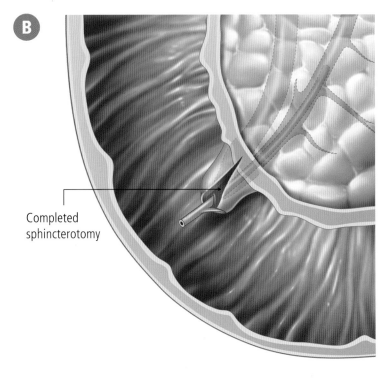

B

Completed
sphincterotomy

Precut over pancreatic duct stent

05 Endoscopic sphincterotomy (EST)

❶ Basic technique

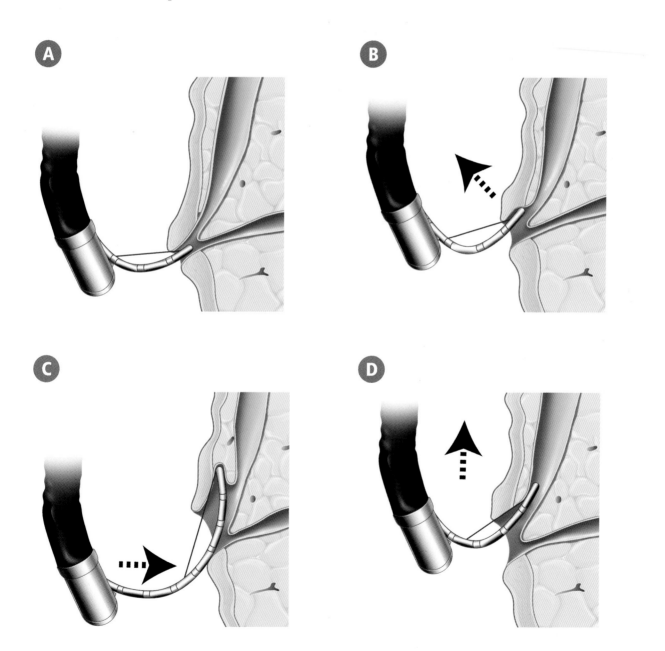

Cannulation using pull-type sphincterotome before EST

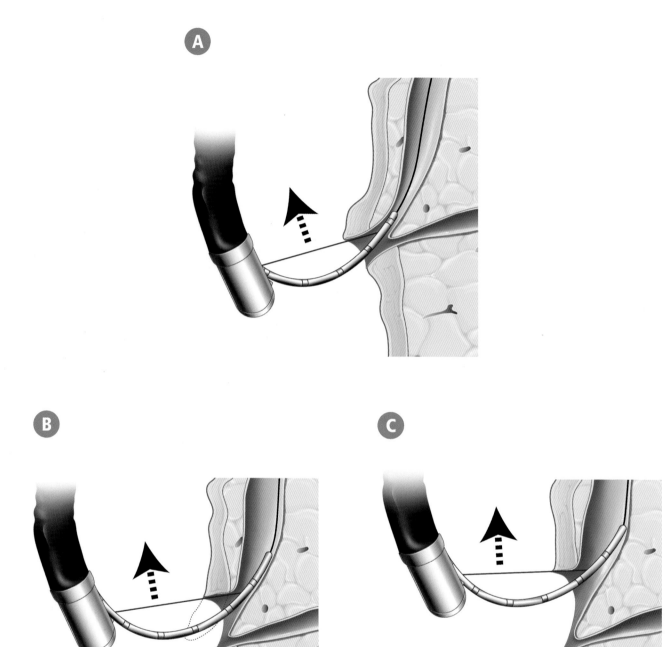

Endoscopic sphincterotomy (EST)

Minimize the contact between wire and mucosa. Proceed with incision in the upward direction.
Direction of incision should be between 11 and 1 o'clock.

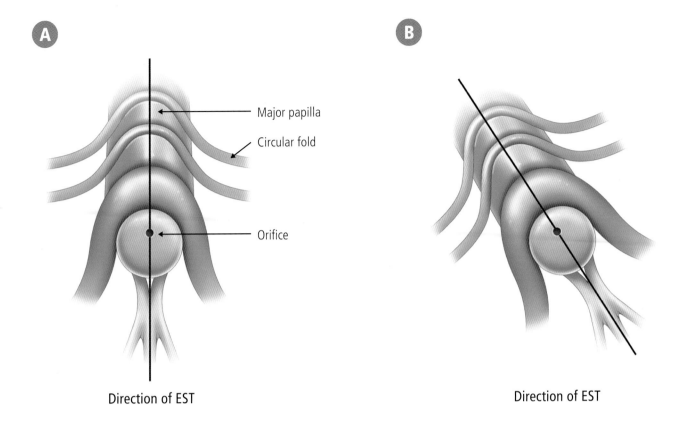

A

Major papilla

Circular fold

Orifice

Direction of EST

B

Direction of EST

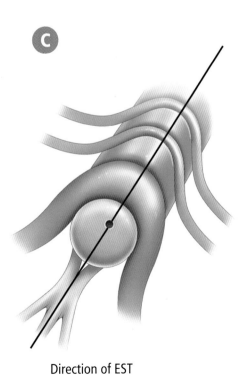

C

Direction of EST

| EST | endoscopic sphincterotomy |

Direction of endoscopic biliary sphincterotomy

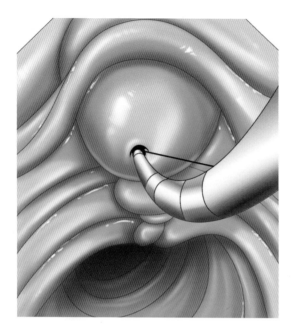
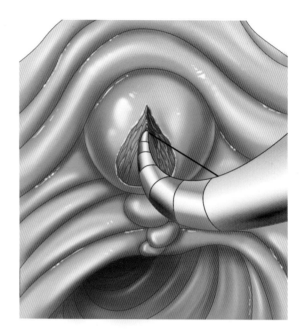
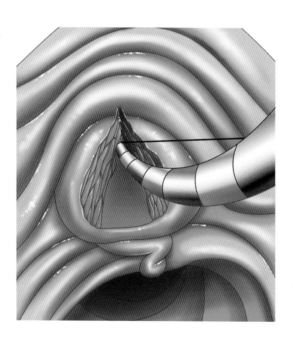
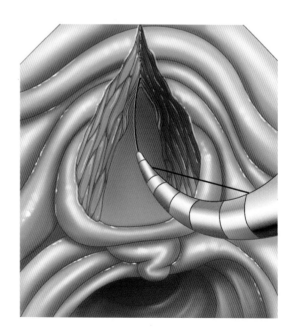

Opening of ampulla as EST proceeds

❷ Advanced technique

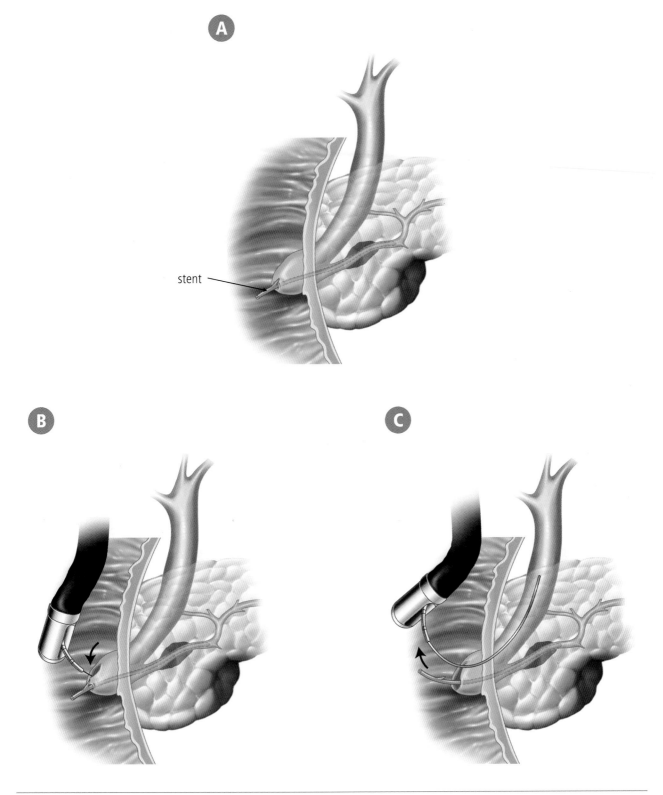

Precut sphincterotomy guided by pancreatic duct stent

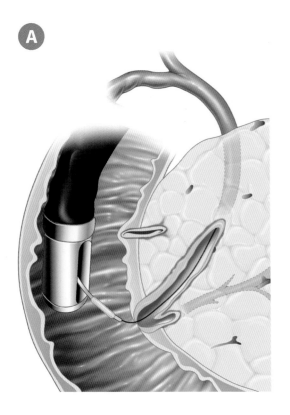

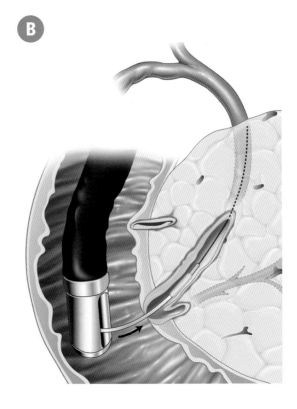

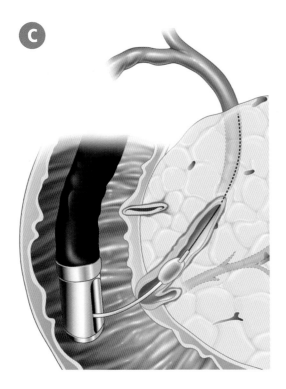

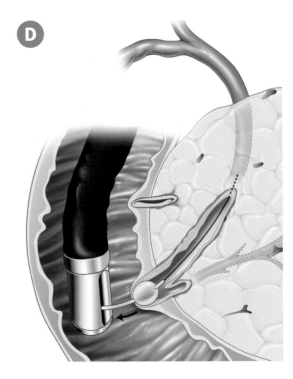

Inflated-balloon-pulling technique for estimating the adequate extent of EST

A) Introducing balloon catheter, B) Inserting balloon catheter into bile duct
C) Fully inflating balloon, D) Pulling inflated balloon catheter toward the duodenal lumen

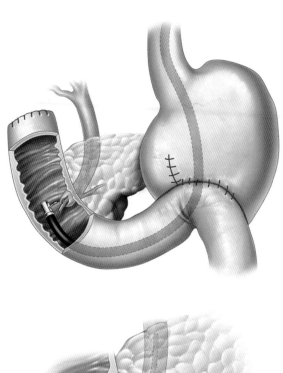

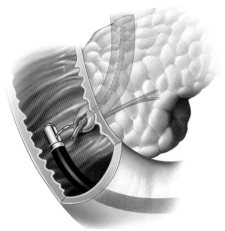

Duodenocope

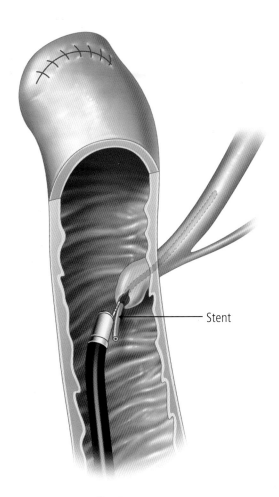

Stent

Gastroscope

EST using needle knife over the stent in Billroth II gastrectomy

❸ Minor papilla sphicterotomy

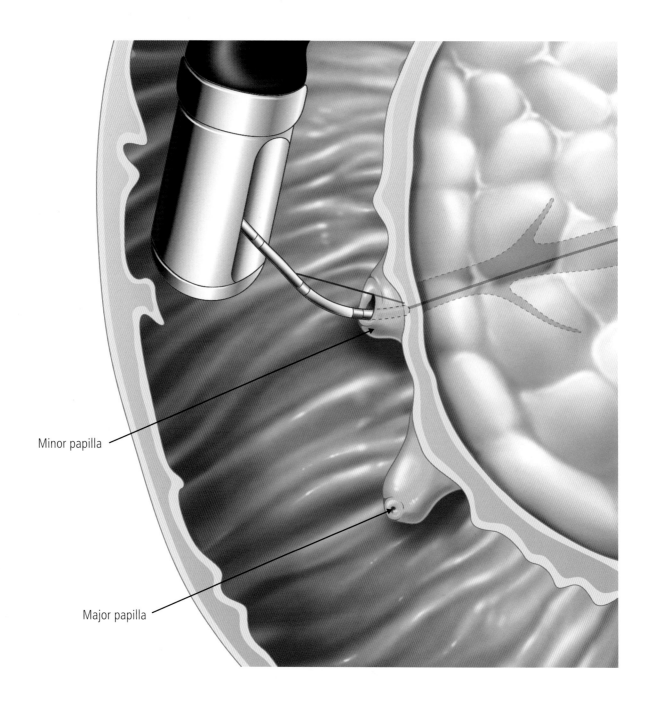

Minor papilla

Major papilla

Minor papilla sphincterotomy

Deep cannulation of minor papilla is important.
Perform EST using pull-type sphincterotome in longitudinal direction (usually towards 10 o'clock direction).

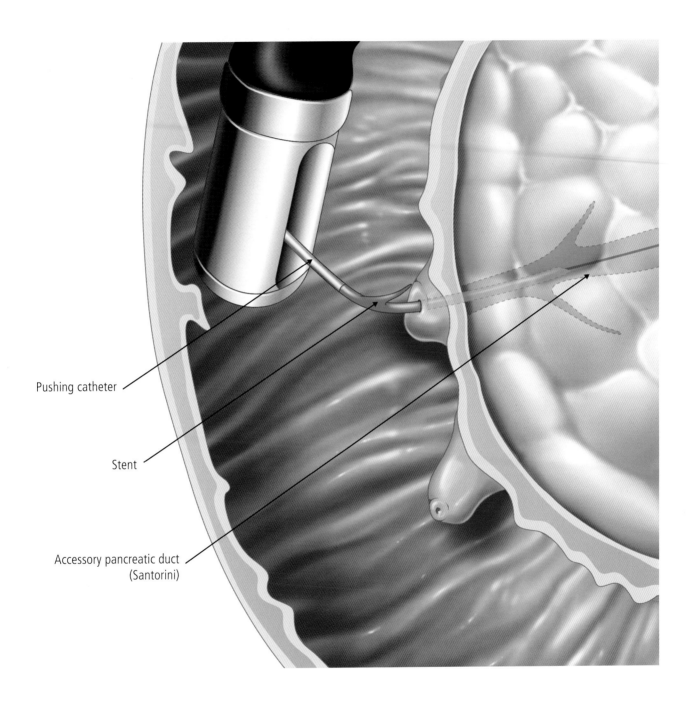

Pushing catheter

Stent

Accessory pancreatic duct
(Santorini)

Insertion of minor papillary stent

06 Drainage

❶ Endoscopic nasobiliary drainage (ENBD)

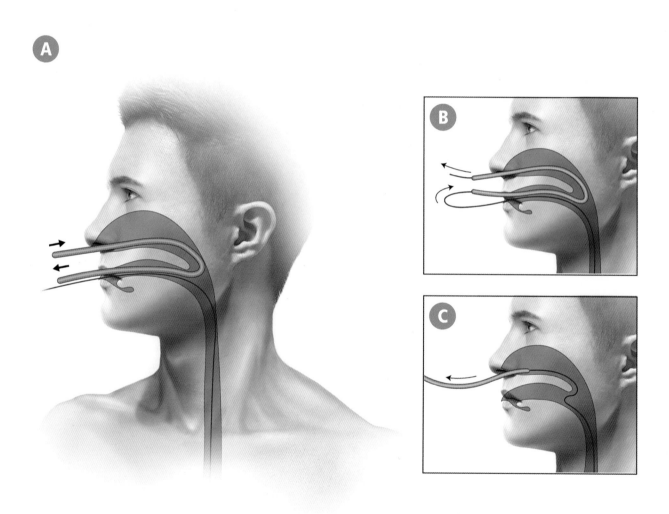

Method of extracting ENBD tube through the nose

❷ Endoscopic retrograde biliary drainage (ERBD)

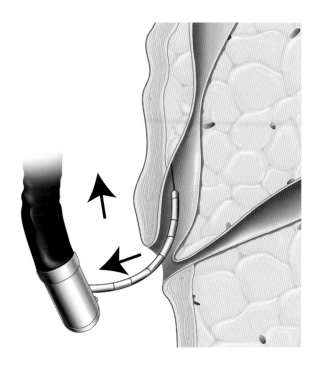

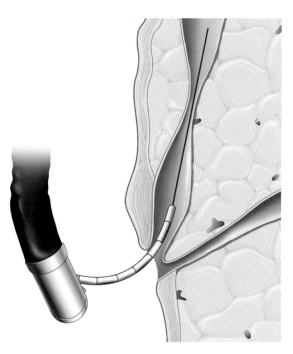

Pull back the scope and catheter to improve the angle for guidewire advancement

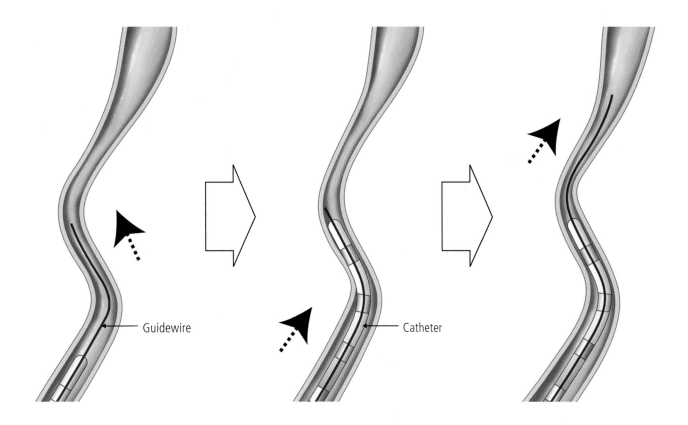

Guidewire

Catheter

Advance through tortuous strictures one bend at a time, first the guidewire and then the catheter

A

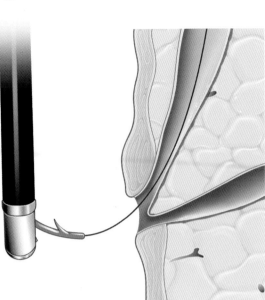

Advance the stent tip until it comes into view

B

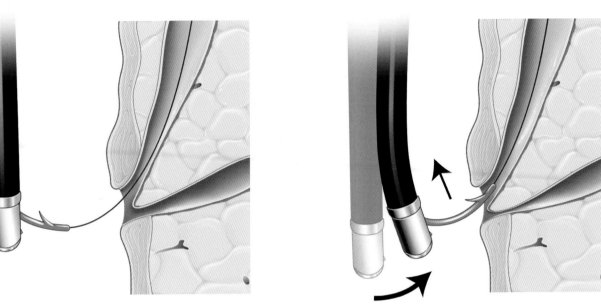

Insert the stent tip into the bile duct by angling
the scope tip up and lifting the elevator

C

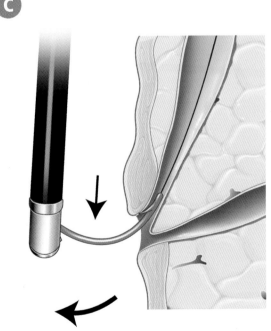

Then back off the scope slightly (angle down),
drop the elevator and advance the stent slightly

D

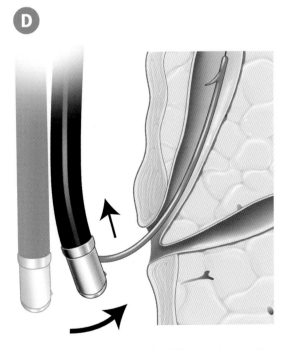

Then push the stent into the bile duct by angling
the scope tip and lifting the elevator

Inserting the plastic biliary stent

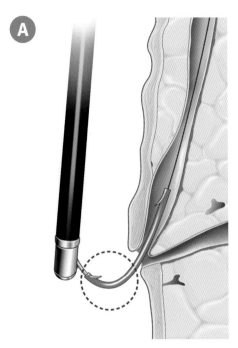

If there is too much stent in the duodenum

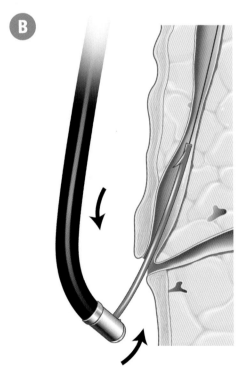

Advance the scope and angle it up to
get the stent straight

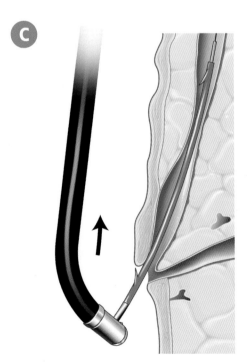

Then pull back on the scope to force
the stent inwards

Getting out of loop trouble

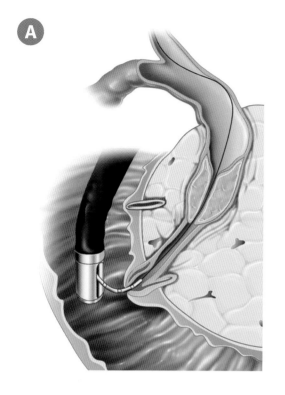

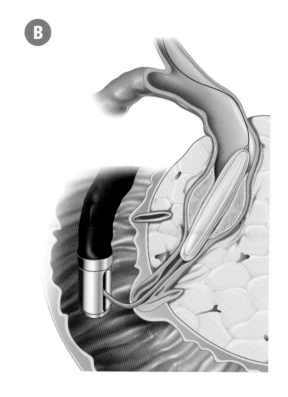

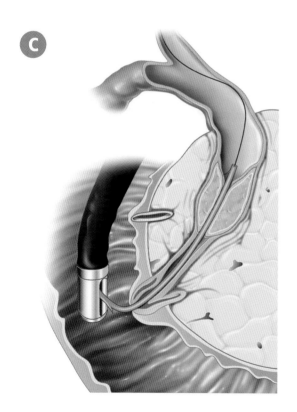

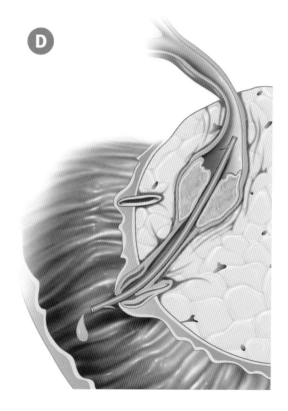

Endoscopic technique for balloon dilation and plastic biliary stent placement

❸ Removal of plastic stent

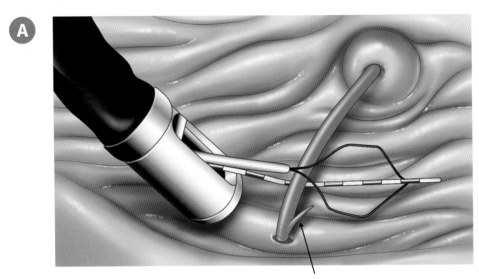

Distally migrated impacted stent

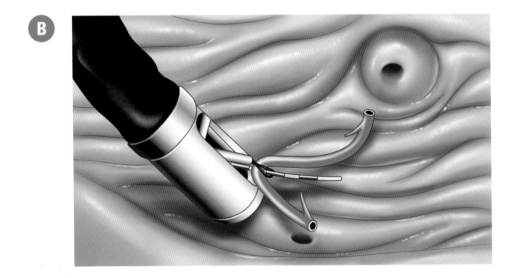

The "lasso" technique for removing a distally migrated stent that had impacted against the contralateral duodenal wall

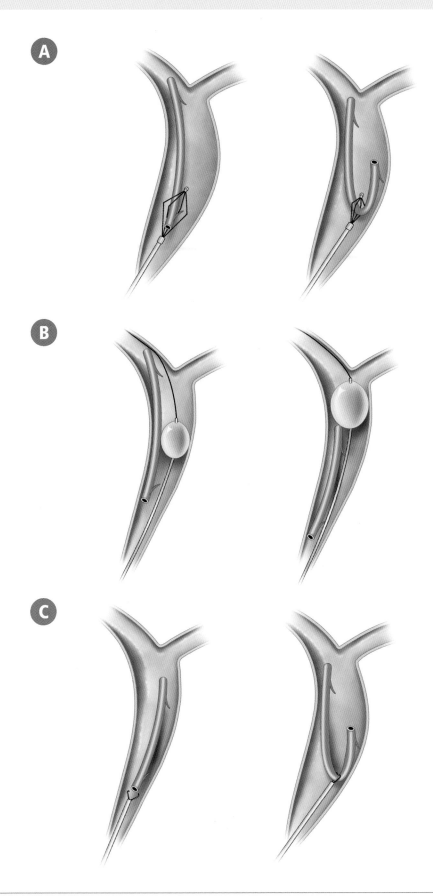

Indirect grasping technique for proximally migrated stent.

A) basket , B) retrieval ballon, C) forcep

❹ Self-expandable metal stent (SEMS)

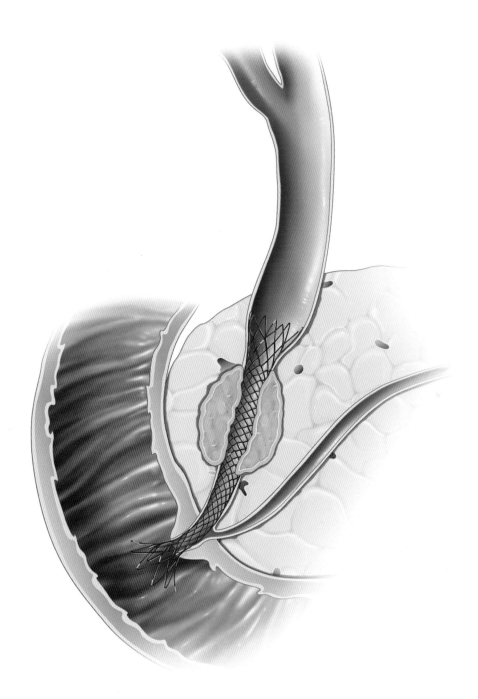

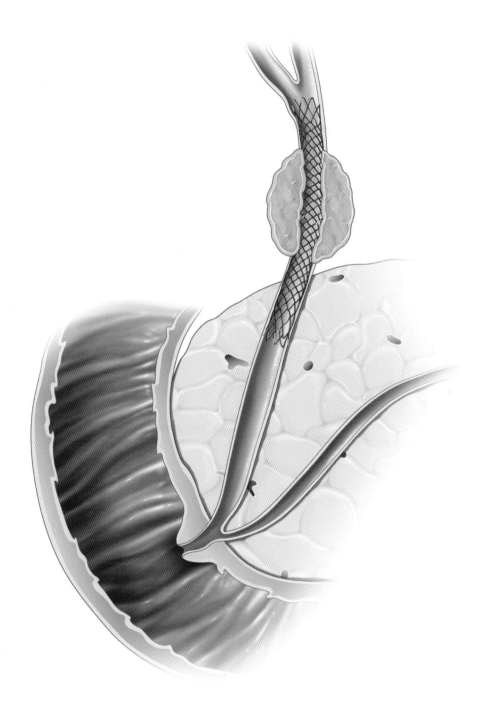

Suprapapillary SEMS

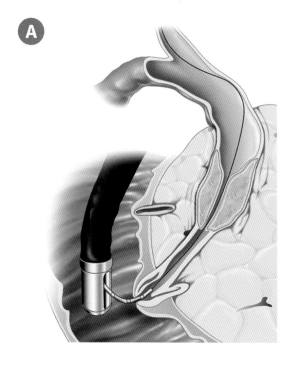

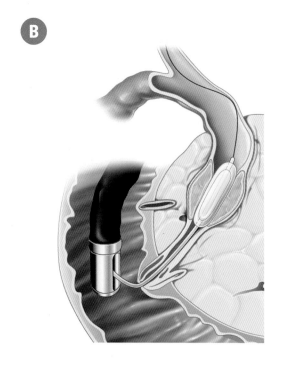

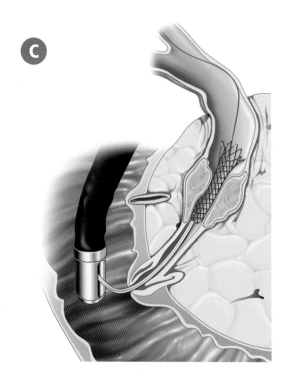

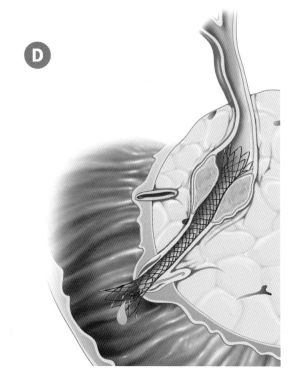

Endoscopic techinque for balloon dilation and SEMS placement

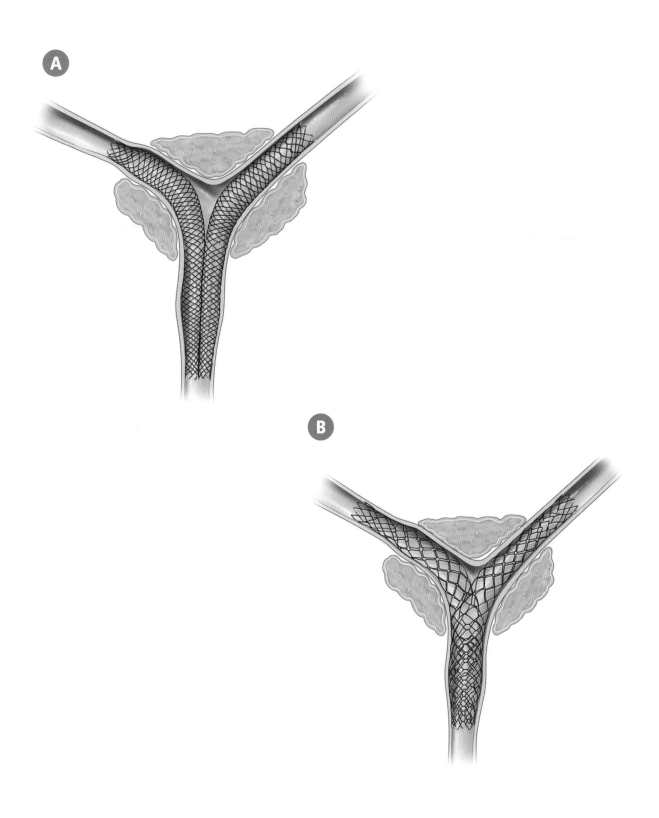

Hilar bilateral SEMS

A) Side-by-side metal stents, B) Stent-in-stent metal stents

❺ Endoscopic retrograde pancreatic drainage (ERPD)

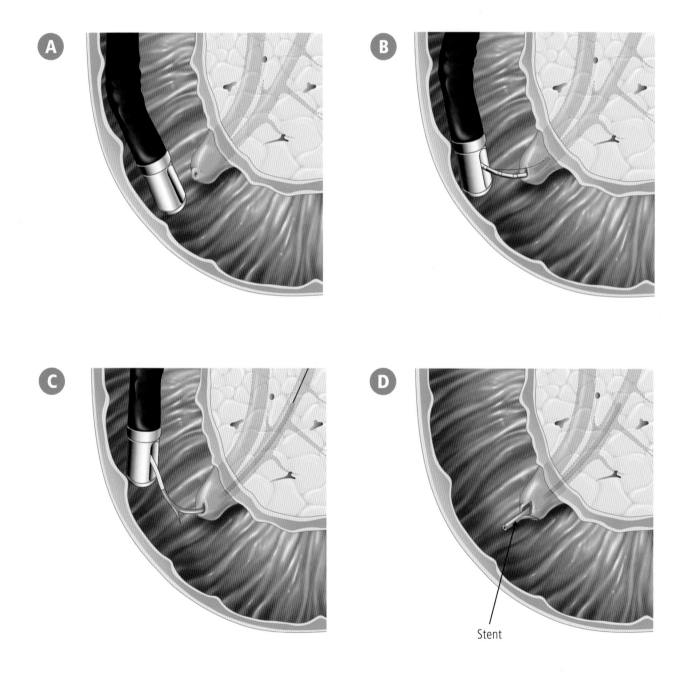

Stent

❻ Pancreatic duct leakage

A

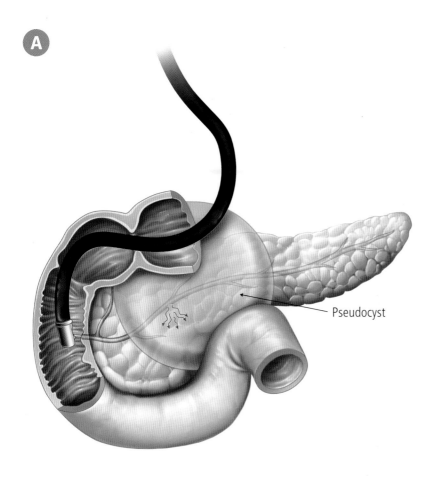

Pseudocyst

B

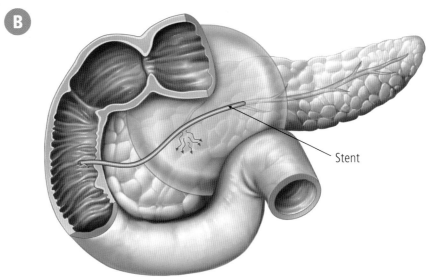

Stent

A) Pancreatic duct leakage
B) Ideal position of pancreatic duct stent placement across the leakage site

07 Stone extraction

❶ Impacted stone in the ampulla of Vater

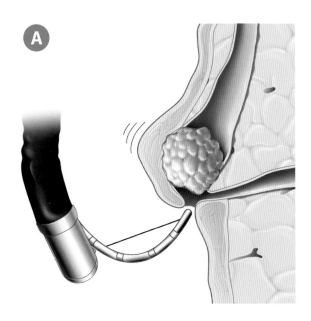

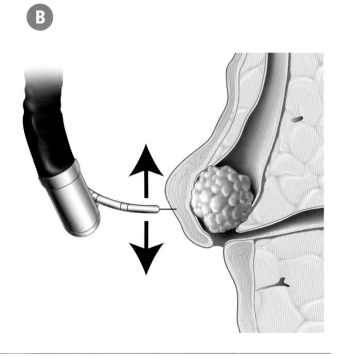

A) A bowed papillotome for cannulating bile duct
B) A needle knife papillotome for incising over the stone

❷ Stone extraction with basket

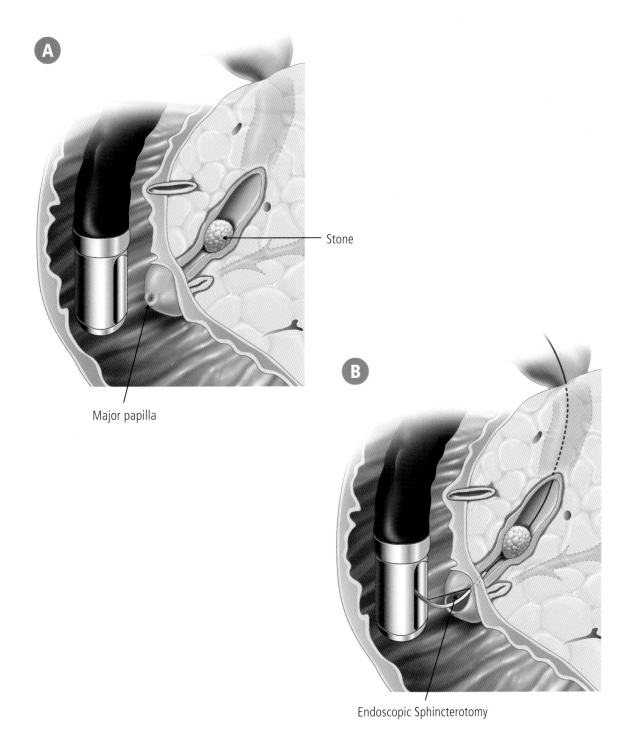

A

Stone

Major papilla

B

Endoscopic Sphincterotomy

Basic technique

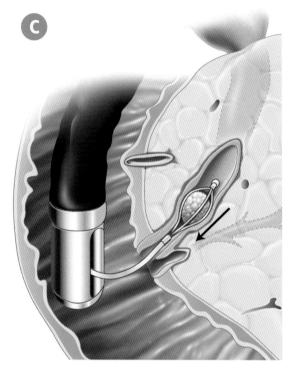

Capturing stone

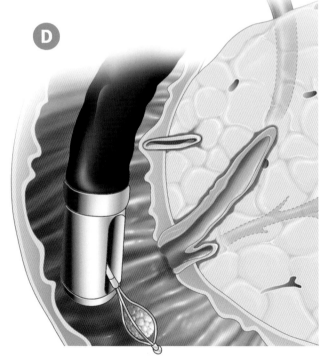

Extracting bile duct stone

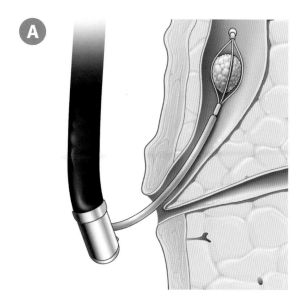

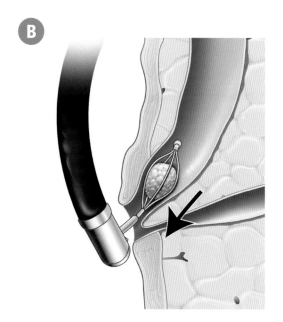

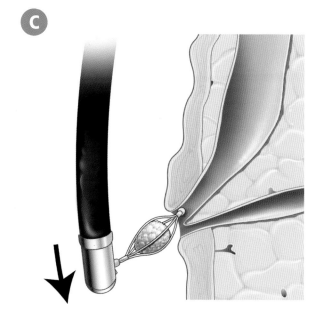

Tips on using basket

Flip-down technique for removing stone

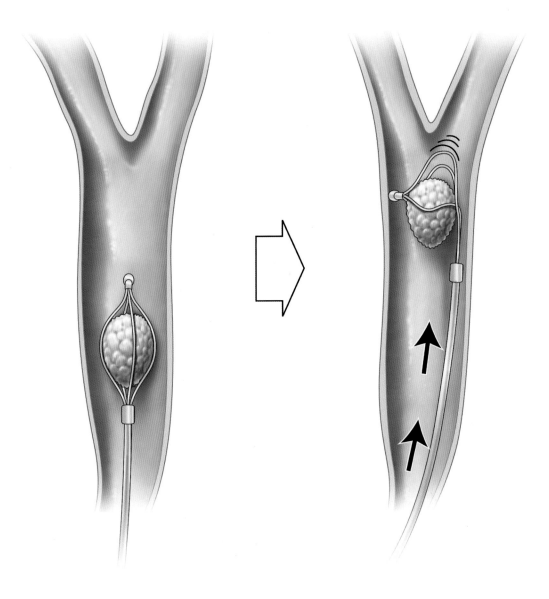

Tips on using basket

Advancing and distorting the basket for releasing the stone

❸ Stone extraction with balloon catheter

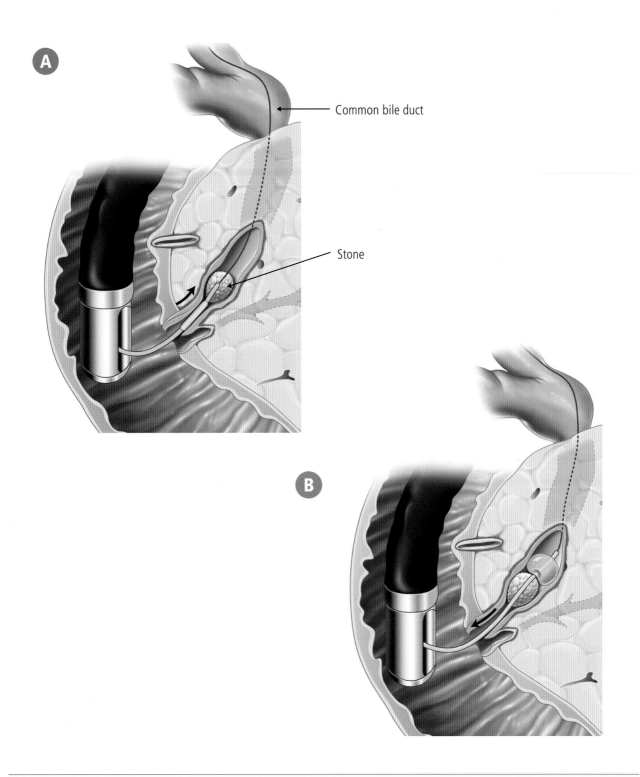

Common bile duct

Stone

Pulling bile duct stone with an inflated balloon catheter

Removing bile duct stone (A, B, C)

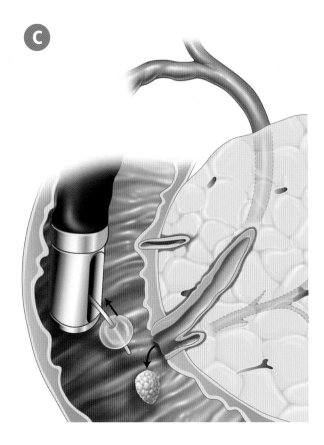

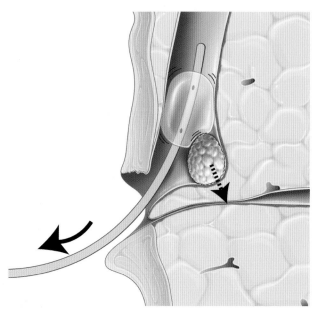

A kind of difficulty with balloon catheter
in extracting bile duct stone

Pulling bile duct stone with an inflated balloon catheter

Removing bile duct stone (A, B, C)

❹ Stone fragmentation (Ⅰ)

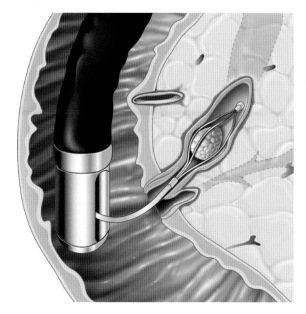

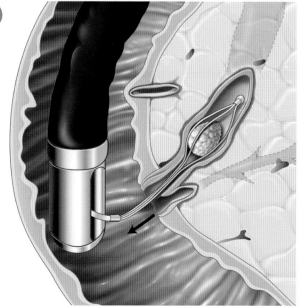

Mechanical lithotripsy with the through-the-scope lithotriptor

A) Capturing bile duct stone, B) Removing basket sheath

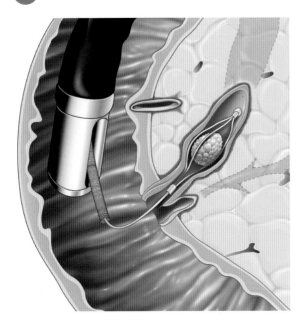

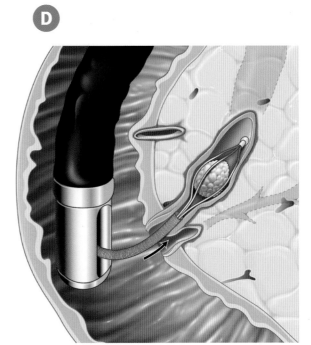

Mechanical lithotripsy with the through-the-scope lithotriptor

C) Introducing metal tube, D) Advancing metal tube

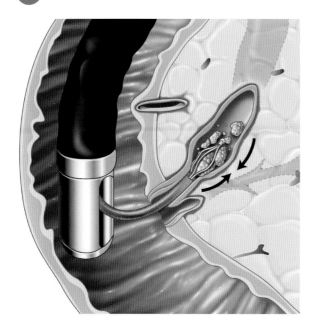

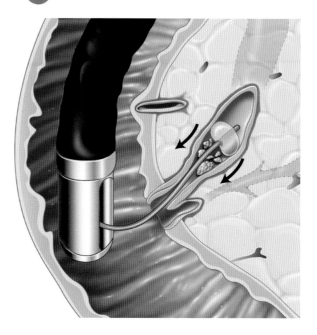

Mechanical lithotripsy with the through-the-scope lithotriptor

E) Crushing bile duct stone, F) Removing fragmented stones with balloon catheter

❹ Stone fragmentation (Ⅱ)

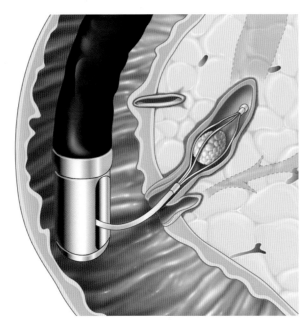

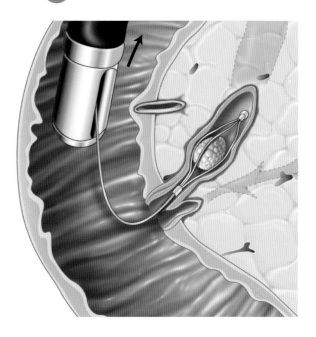

Emergency (Rescue) lithotripsy

A) Capturing bile duct stone, B) Withdrawing duodenoscope

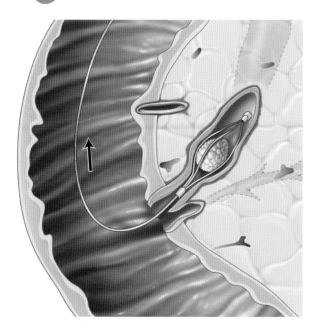

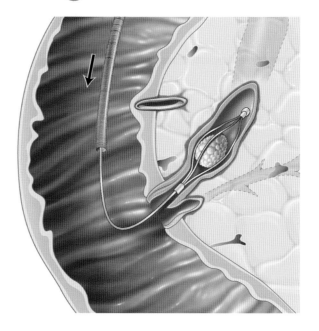

Emergency (Rescue) lithotripsy

C) Removing basket sheath, D) Introducing metal tube

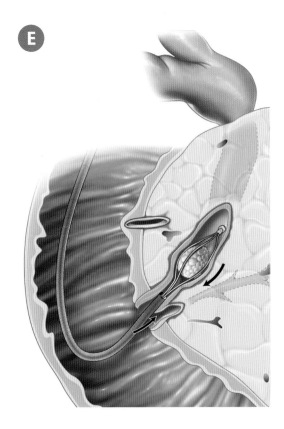

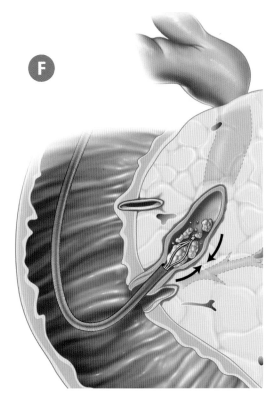

Emergency (Rescue) lithotripsy

E) Advancing metal tube, F) Crushing bile duct stone

❹ Stone fragmentation (Ⅲ)

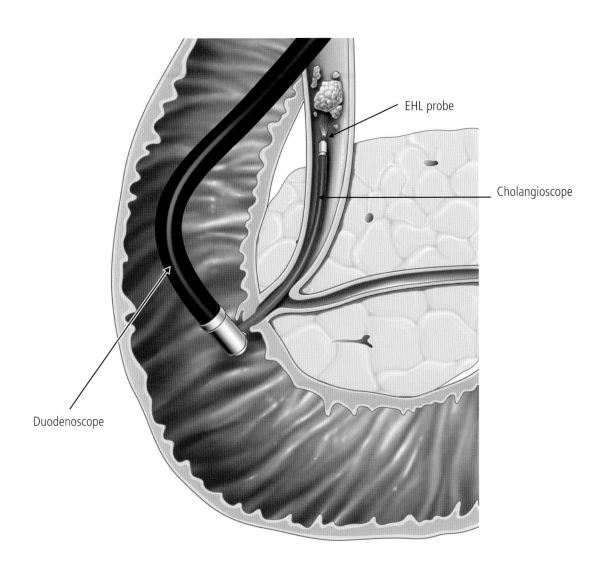

EHL probe

Cholangioscope

Duodenoscope

Electrohydraulic lithotripsy (EHL) with peroral cholangioscope

❹ Stone fragmentation (Ⅳ)

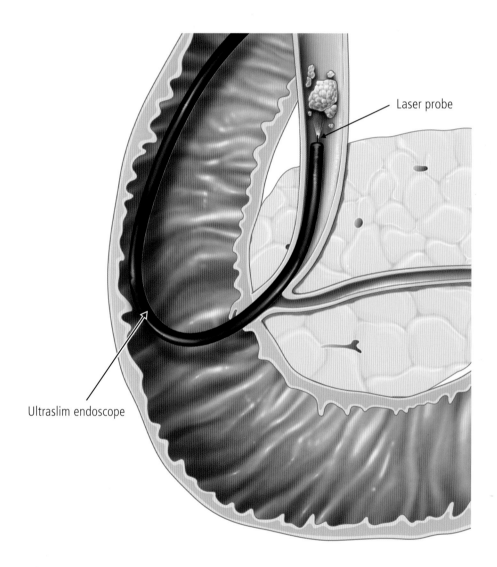

Laser probe

Ultraslim endoscope

Laser lithotripsy under direct peroral cholangioscope

❺ Pancreatic duct stone

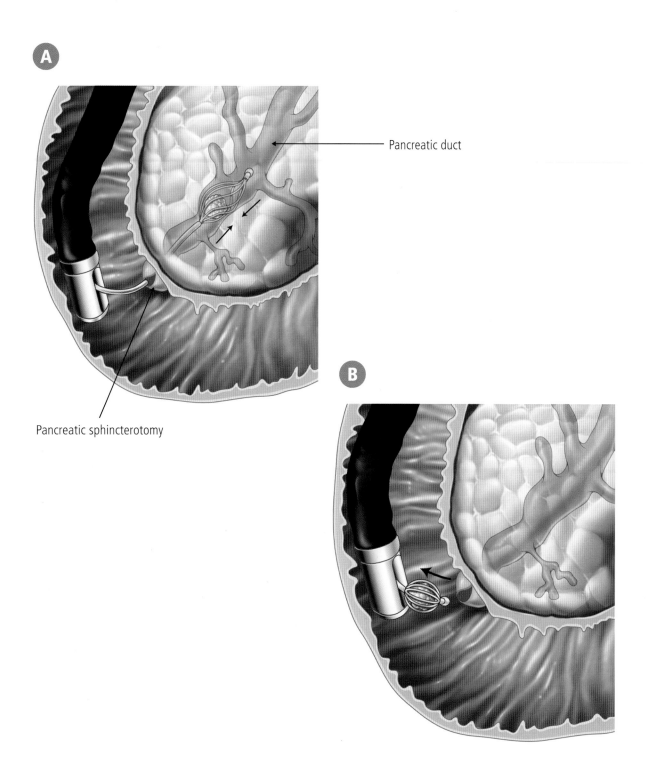

A

Pancreatic duct

Pancreatic sphincterotomy

B

Extraction of parcreatic duct stone using basket

08 Papillectomy

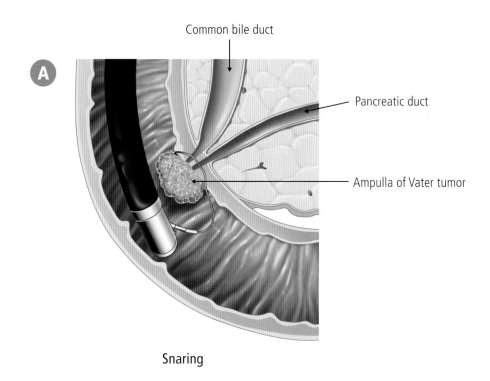

Common bile duct

Pancreatic duct

Ampulla of Vater tumor

Snaring

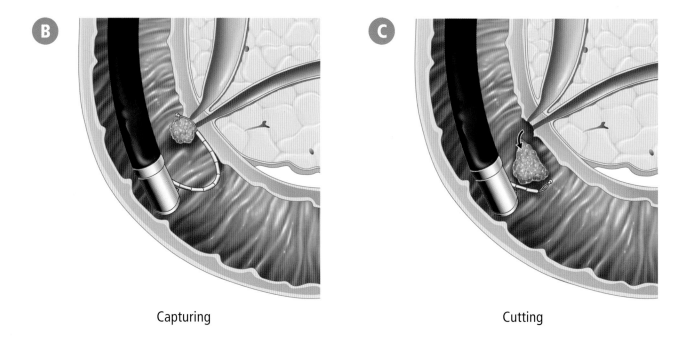

Capturing

Cutting

09 Rescue methods of ERCP

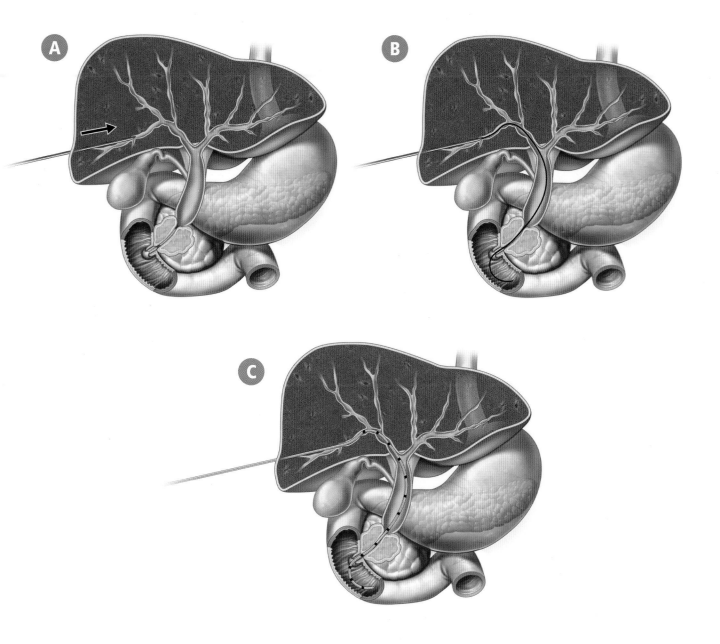

Percutaneous transhepatic biliary drainage (PTBD)

A) Needle puncture of dilated intrahepatic bile duct under image guidance
B) Guidewire insertion through the needle into biliary system
C) Placement of biliary drainage catheter with multiple side holes

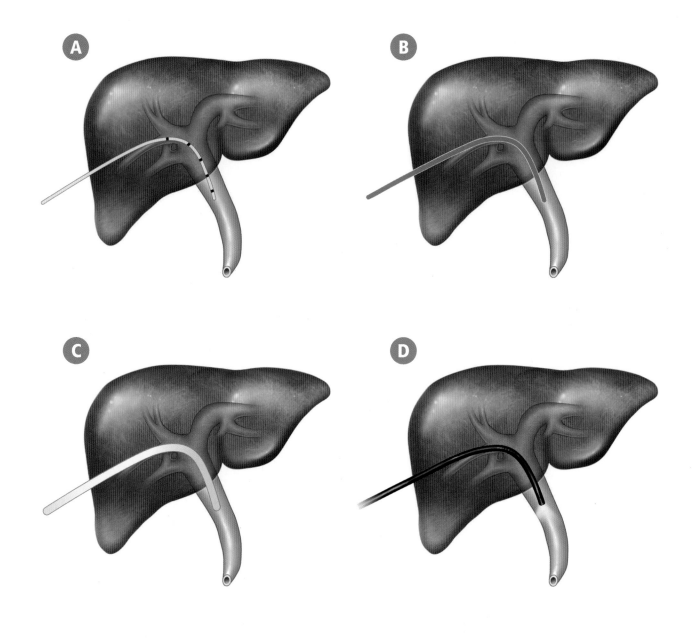

Percutaneous transhepatic cholangioscopy (PTCS)

A) Percutaneous transhepatic biliary drainage catheter was placed on the dilated intrahepatic bile duct (6-8fr)
B) Percutaneous transhepatic tract dilation up to 10-12Fr
C) Percutaneous transhepatic tract dilation up to 16-20Fr
D) Cholanigioscope entered into through the dilated tract

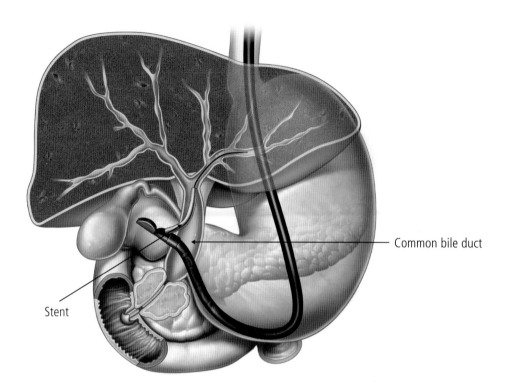

Common bile duct

Stent

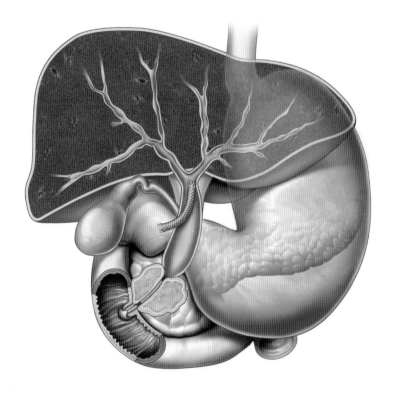

EUS guided choledochoduodenostomy (EUS-CDS)

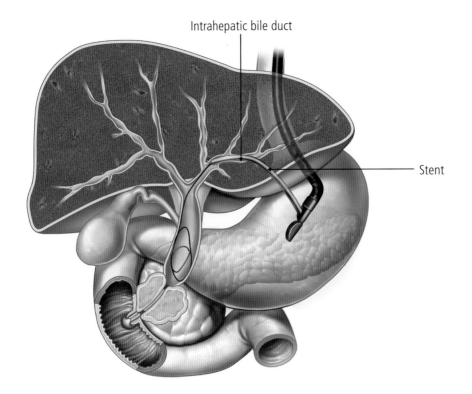

Intrahepatic bile duct

Stent

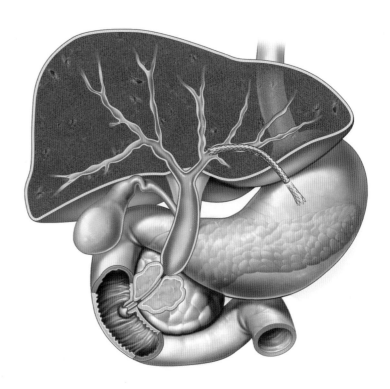

EUS guided hepaticogastrostomy (EUS-HGS)

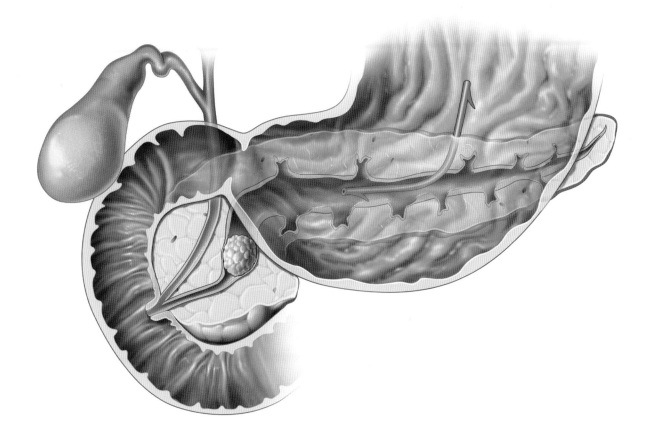

EUS guided pancreatic duct drainage

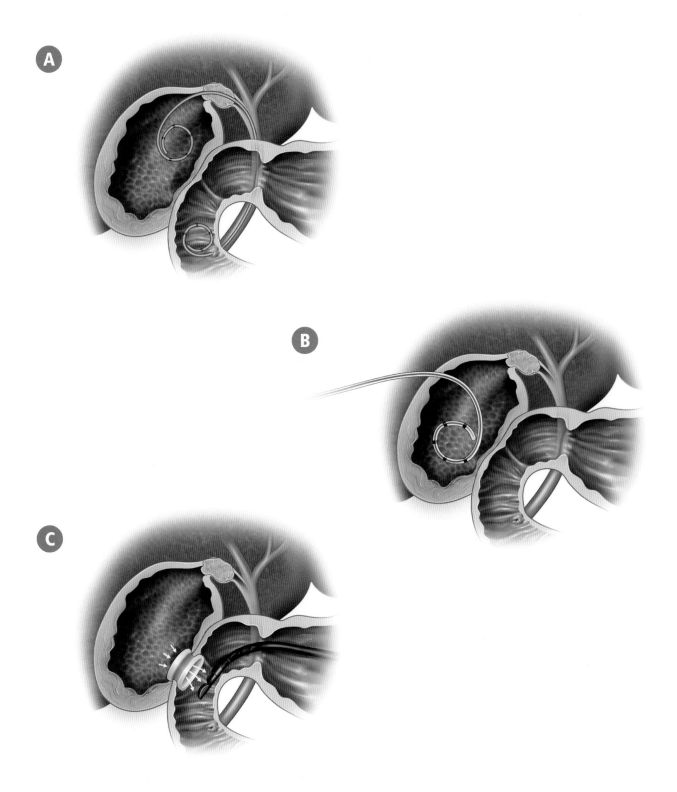

Gallbladder drainage
A) Endoscopic retrograde gallbladder drainage (ERGBD)
B) Percutaneous transhepatic gallbladder drainage (PTGBD)
C) EUS guided gallbladder drainage (EUS-GBD)

VI

ERCP Accessories

01 Guidewire

Guidewire

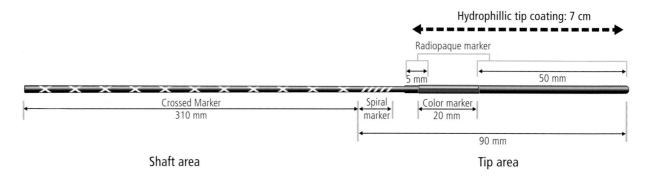

Hydrophillic tip coating: 7 cm

Radiopaque marker

5 mm

50 mm

Crossed Marker
310 mm

Spiral marker

Color marker
20 mm

90 mm

Shaft area

Tip area

Composition of tip

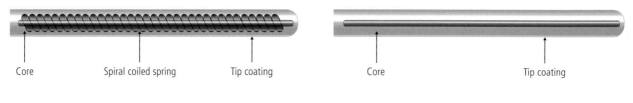

Core

Spiral coiled spring

Tip coating

Spiral coiled spring wire type

Core

Tip coating

Monofilament coated wire type

Different shapes of tip

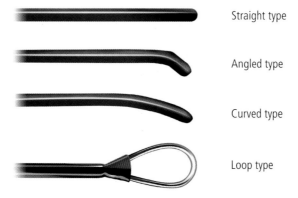

Straight type

Angled type

Curved type

Loop type

Table 1. Basic characteristics of the currently available ERCP guidewires in Korea*

Manufacturer	Commercial name	Diameter (inch)	Length (cm)	Core material	Sheath material	Tip length (cm)	Tip core material	Spiral coiled spring	Tip coating	Shape of tip
Boston Scientific	Jagwire™	0.035	200, 260, 450	Nitinol	PTFE	5	Tungsten	No	Hydrophilic polyurethane	Straight/Angled
		0.025	260, 450	Nitinol	PTFE	5	Tungsten	No	Hydrophilic polyurethane	Straight/Angled
	Hydra Jagwire™	0.035	260, 450	Nitinol	PTFE	5	Tungsten	No	Hydrophilic polyurethane	Straight/Angled
	Dreamwire™	0.035	260, 450	Nitinol	PTFE	10	Tungsten	No	Hydrophilic polyurethane	Straight/Angled
	Jagwire™ Revolution	0.025	260, 450, 500	Nitinol	PTFE	5	Tungsten	No	Hydrophilic polyurethane	Straight/Angled
Cook Endoscopy	Fusion Loop Tip™	0.035	205, 260, 480	Nitinol	PTFE	0.4	Platinum	Yes	ETFE	Fixed loop
	Tracer Metro Direct®	0.035	260, 480	Nitinol	PTFE	5	Platinum	Yes	Hydrophilic polyurethane	Straight/ Angled
		0.025	260, 480	Nitinol	PTFE	5	Platinum	Yes	Hydrophilic polyurethane	Straight
		0.021	260, 480	Nitinol	PTFE	5	Platinum	Yes	Hydrophilic polyurethane	Straight
	Acrobat II®	0.035	205, 260, 450	Nitinol	PTFE	4	Platinum	Yes	Hydrophilic polyurethane	Straight/Angled
		0.025	260, 450	Nitinol	PTFE	4	Platinum	Yes	Hydrophilic polyurethane	Straight/Angled
	Road Runner®	0.018	260, 480	Nitinol	PTFE	3	Platinum	No	n/a	Straight/Angled
Medwork	gSlider	0.033	450	Nitinol	PTFE	5.5	Nitinol	No	Hydrophilic polyurethane	Straight/Angled
MTW Endoskopie	Platin star	0.025	460	Nitinol	PTFE	7	Platinum	No	Hydrophilic polyurethane	Straight
		0.035	400	Nitinol	PTFE	5	Platinum	No	Hydrophilic polyurethane	Straight/Curved
	Snap-tip	0.025	460	Nitinol	PTFE	5	Platinum	No	Hydrophilic polyurethane	Straight
		0.035	460	Nitinol	PTFE	5	Platinum	No	Hydrophilic polyurethane	Straight
	Grip-wire	0.035	460	Nitinol	PTFE	8.3	Platinum	No	Hydrophilic polyurethane	Straight/Curved
Olympus	VisiGlide 2	0.025	270, 450	Nitinol	Fluorine coating polyethylene	7	Confidential	Yes	Hydrophilic PTFE	Straight/Angled
Taewoong Medical	Optimos™	0.035	260, 450	Nitinol	PTFE	5.5	Nitinol	No	Hydrophilic polyurethane	Straight/Angled
		0.025	260, 450	Nitinol	PTFE	5.5	Nitinol	No	Hydrophilic polyurethane	Straight/Angled

* Some items (especially, tip coating materials) are not accurate due to the confidentiality of the company.
ETFE, Ethylenetetrafluoroethylene; PTFE, Polytetrafluoroethylene;

02 Cannula

ERCP cannula

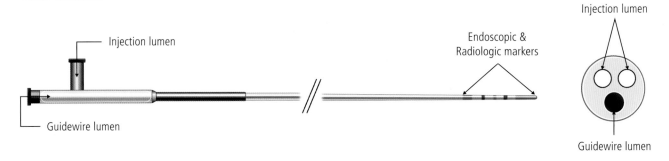

Type of ERCP cannula

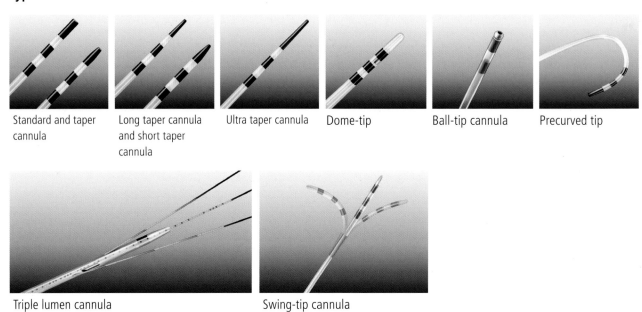

Standard and taper cannula | Long taper cannula and short taper cannula | Ultra taper cannula | Dome-tip | Ball-tip cannula | Precurved tip

Triple lumen cannula   Swing-tip cannula

Table 2. Basic characteristics of the currently available ERCP cannulas (catheters) in Korea

Manufacturer	Commercial name	Length (cm)	Distal tip (Fr)	Tip shape	Available guidewire (Inch)	Separate injection lumen	Special characteristics
Boston Scientific	Contour™ ERCP Cannulas	210	5.0	Standard	0.035	X	
		210	5.0	Tapered	0.035	X	
		210	5.0	Ultra-Tapered	0.025	X	
		210	5.0	5-4-3	0.018	X	
		210	5.0	Ball-Tip	0.035	X	

Manufacturer	Commercial name	Length (cm)	Distal tip (Fr)	Tip shape	Available guidewire (Inch)	Separate injection lumen	Special characteristics
Boston Scientific	Rapid exchange XL Cannula	195	5.5	Tapered	0.035	X	
	RX ERCP Cannulas	210	5.0	Standard	0.035	X	
		210	5.0	Tapered	0.035	X	
		210	5.0	Ball-Tip	0.035	X	
	Tandem™ XL Triple-Lumen ERCP Cannula	200	5.5	Tapered	0.035	O	Separated lumen
Cook Endoscopy	Classic						
	ERCP-1-BT	200	5.5	Metal radiopaque bullet	0.035	X	
	Huibregtse-Katon®						
	ERCP-1-HKB	200	5.5	Metal Ball tip	0.035	X	Metal tip
	Glo-Tip®						
	GT-1-T	200	5.5 → 4.5	Taper	0.035	X	
	GT-1-ST	200	5.5 → 3.5	Short taper	0.025	X	
	GT-1-LT	200	5.5 → 3.5	Long taper	0.021	X	
	GT-1-UT	200	5.5 → 4.0	Ultra taper	0.035	X	
	GT-5-4-3	200	5.0 → 4.0 → 3.0	Precurved, graduated taper	0.018	X	
	Glo-Tip II®						
	GT-2-T	200	6.0	Standard Dome-shaped tip	0.035	O	Double lumen (separated lumen)
	GT-2-T-RB	200	6.0	Standard Dome-shaped tip	0.035	O	Double lumen (separated lumen) Radiopaque Band
	Fusion®						
	FS-GT-2	200	6.0	Standard Dome-shaped tip	0.035	O	
	Fusion® OMNI™						
	FS-GT-OMNI	200	7.0	Standard Dome-shaped tip	0.035	O	Breakthrough channel technology
MTW Endoskopie	ERCP-catheter with integrated mandrin	215	5.4 / 4.8	Filiform	0.035 / 0.025	X	
		215	5.4 / 4.8	Filiform, with Metal Ring Inside	0.035 / 0.025	X	
		215	5.4 / 4.8	With round metal tip	0.035 / 0.025	X	Metal tip
		215	5.4 / 4.8	Bottle shaped metal tip	0.035 / 0.025	X	Metal tip
		215	5.4 / 4.8	Conical metal tip	0.035 / 0.025	X	Metal tip
Medwork	ERCP-Cannulas	205	5.4	Tapered	0.035	X	Single lumen
		204	5.55	Tapered	0.035	O	Double lumen
Olympus	StarTipV™ with Soft/Stiff	195	4.0	Standard	0.035	X	
		195	4.0 / 3.5	Taper	0.035 / 0.025	X	
		195	4.5 / 4.0 / 3.5	Short taper	0.035 / 0.035 / 0.025	X	
		195	3.5 / 3.0	Long taper	0.025	X	
		195	6.0	Metal Ball	0.035	X	Metal tip
	StarTip2V™	170	4.5	Short taper	0.035	O	Double Lumen
	X-PressV™ with Soft/Stiff	195	2.5	Slit	0.035	X	
	SwingTip™	195	4.0	Bendable Taper	0.035	X	Pull: 85° Push: 20°

03 Sphincterotome

Sphincterotome

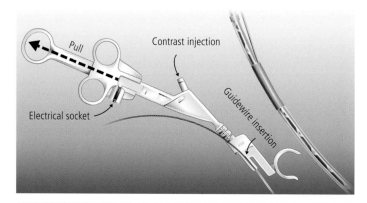

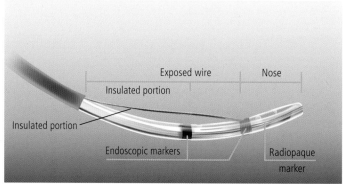

Types of sphincterotome

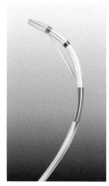

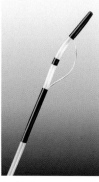

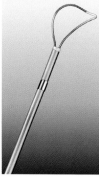

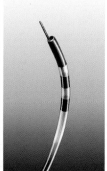

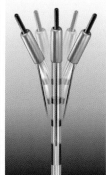

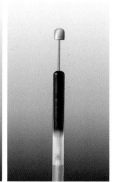

Pull type sphincterotome

Push type sphincterotome

Reverse type sphincterotome

Needle type sphincterotome

Rotatable sphincterotome

Isolated-tip needle knife

Table 3. Basic characteristics of the currently available ERCP sphincterotomes in Korea

Manufacturer	Commercial name	Type	Tip length (mm)	Cut-wire type	Cut-wire length (mm)	Safe wire insulation	Tip diameter (Fr)	Guidewire (Inch)	Special characteristics
Boston Scientific	Autotome™ RX Cannulating Sphincterotome	Pull type	5	Monofilament	20 / 30	X	3.9 / 4.4 / 4.9	0.025 / 0.035	Rotating tip
	UltraTome™ RX Cannulating Sphincterotome	Pull type	5	Monofilament	20 / 30	X	4.9	0.035	
	TRUEtome™ Cannulating Sphincterotome	Pull type	5	Monofilament	20 / 30	X	3.9 / 4.4 / 4.9	0.025 / 0.035	Rotating tip
	UltraTome™ Double-Lumen Sphincterotome	Pull type	5 / 20	Monofilament	20 / 30	X	5.5	0.035	Double lumen
	UltraTome™ XL Triple-Lumen Sphincterotome	Pull type	5 / 20	Monofilament	20 / 30	X	5.5	0.035	Triple lumen
	MicroKnife XL Triple-Lumen Needle knife	Needle type	n/a	Monofilament	7	n/a	5.5	0.035	Triple lumen
Cook Endoscopy	Tri-Tome PC® Triple lumen Sphincterotome with DomeTip® (Protector™)	Pull type	5	Monofilament	25	O	7.0	0.035	
	Tri-Tome PC® Triple lumen Sphincterotome with DomeTip®	Pull type	5	Monofilament / Braided	20 / 25 / 30	X	7.0	0.035	
	Cotton CannulaTome II® Precurved Double Lumen Sphincterotome with DomeTip® (Protector™)	Pull type	5	Monofilament	25	O	6.0	0.035	
	Fusion® OMNI™ Sphincterotome with DomeTip®	Pull type	5	Monofilament	25	X	5.5 / 7.0	0.021 / 0.035	Breakthrough channel technology
	Billroth II Sphincterotome	Push type	n/a	Braided	20 / 30	X	6.0 → 5.0	0.035	
	Fusion® Needle knife	Needle type	n/a	Monofilament	4	n/a	6.0	0.035	Adjustable Cutting Wire Length
MTW Endoskopie	Papillotome, filiform	Pull type	5	Monofilament	20 / 30	X	4.8	0.035	
	Papillotome, Precut	Pull type	2	Monofilament	20	X	4.8	0.035	2 mm tip length
	Papillotome for B-II-Stomach	Push type	5	Monofilament	20	X	6.9	0.035	
	Papillotome, Needle	Needle type	6	Monofilament	6	n/a	4.5	0.035	6 mm tip length
	Iso-Tome	Needle type	10	Monofilament	10	O	4.5	n/a	Insulated tip
Medwork	AXS_tome Papillotomes (2 Lumen)	Pull type	5	Monofilament / Braided	20 / 25 / 30	X	5.1 / 7	0.021 / 0.035	
		Needle type	n/a	Monofilament	6	n/a	7	0.035	
		Push type	5	Braided	20	X	7	0.021	
	AXS_tome Papillotomes (3 Lumen)	Pull type	5	Monofilament / Braided	20 / 25 / 30	O	7.5	0.035	
		Needle type	n/a	Monofilament	6	n/a	7.5	0.035	
Olympus	CleverCut3V™	Pull type	2 / 3 / 7	Monofilament	15 / 20 / 25 / 30	O	3.9 / 4.4	0.025 / 0.035	Pre-curved design
	Reusable Stabilizer S.-Push/Pull Type	Pull/ Push type	6	Monofilament	15	X	4.5	0.035	For Billroth II, Roux-en-Y
	NeedleCut3V™	Needle type	n/a	Monofilament	5	O/X	5.0	0.035	
Taewoong	Optimos™ Sphincterotome	Pull type	6	Monofilament	20 / 25 / 30	O	5.0	0.025 / 0.035	Pre-curved design

04 Dilating catheter

Dilating catheter

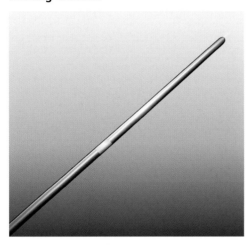
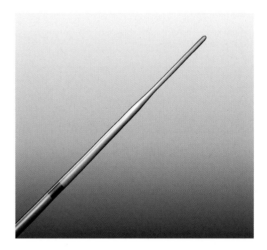

Balloon dilator

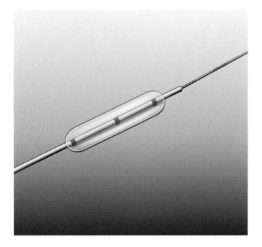

Stent retriever

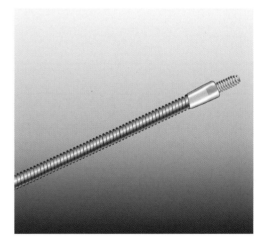

Table 4. **Basic characteristics of the currently available ERCP dilating catheters in Korea**

Manufacturer	Commercial name	Type	Size	Tapered tip length (cm)	Total length (cm)	Balloon length (cm)	Guidewire (Inch)	Special characteristics
Boston Scientific	Hurricane Rx biliary balloon dilators	Balloon dilator	4, 6, 8, 10 mm	0.6	180	2, 4	0.035	Separate guidewire lumen designed for rapid device exchange
	CRE PRO Wire guided Esophageal/ Pyloric/ Biliary Balloon Dilatation Catheters	Balloon dilator	6-7-8, 8-9-10, 10-11-12, 12-13.5-15, 15-16.5-18, 18-19-20 mm		180 / 240	5.5	0.035	
Cook Endoscopy	Soehendra biliary dilation catheters	Dilating catheter	4-6, 4-7, 5-8.5, 6-9, 6-10, 7-11.5 Fr	3	200	n/a	0.035	
	Fusion Titan biliary dilation balloon	Balloon dilator	4, 6, 8, 10 mm	0.8 (Max)	190	4	0.035	
	Fusion biliary dilation balloon	Balloon dilator	4, 6, 8, 10 mm	n/a	188	3	0.035	
	Hercules 3 stage Wire guided balloon	Balloon dilator	8-9-10, 10-11-12, 12-13.5-15, 15-16.5-18, 18-19-20 mm	n/a	240	5.5	0.035	
	Soehendra stent retriever	Stent retriever	5, 7, 8.5, 10, 11.5 Fr		180	n/a	0.035 (5 Fr: 0.021)	Screw tip This device is used to remove plastic stents
Olympus	MaxPass biliary balloon dilators	Balloon dilator	4, 6 mm		180	2, 4	0.035	
			8 mm		180	3	0.035	

05 Stone extraction basket

Types of basket catheter

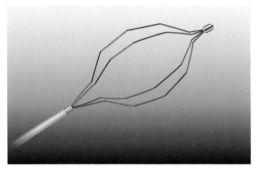

Basic four-wire basket

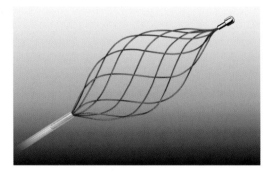

Eight-wire twisted basket

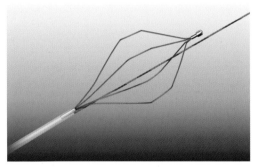

Guidewire-assisted basket

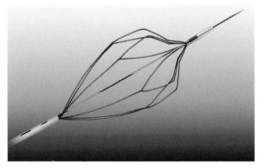

Eight-wire and guidewire-assisted basket

Table 5. Basic characteristics of the currently available stone extraction baskets in Korea

Manufacturer	Commercial name	Basket type	Wire type	Wire material	Wire number	Opening width (mm)	Working length (cm)	Lithotriptor compatable	Special characteristics
Boston Scientific	Trapezoid RX Wire-guided Retrieval Basket	Dormia	Monofilament	Stainless steel	4	15, 20, 25, 30	210	O	Guidewire assisted Compatible with Alliance II Lithotripsy System
Cook Endoscopy	Fusion Lithotripsy Extraction Basket	Dormia	Monofilament	Stainless steel	4	20, 30	208	O	Guidewire assisted
	The Web Extraction Basket	Dormia	Monofilament	Stainless steel /Nitinol	4	15, 20, 25, 30	220	△ (rescue)	
	The Web II Double Lumen Extraction Basket	Fogarty	Monofilament	Stainless steel /Nitinol	4	20	200	X	Guidewire assisted
	Memory Basket 5 FR Soft Wire	Dormia	Monofilament	Stainless steel /Nitinol	4	15, 20	200	X	
	Memory Basket Eight Wire	Spiral	Monofilament	Nitinol	8	20, 30	200	X	
	Memory II Double Lumen Extraction Basket	Spiral	Monofilament	Nitinol	8	20, 30	200	X	Guidewire assisted
Medwork	Stone extraction baskets	Dormia	Monofilament	Stainless steel	4	15, 25, 30, 35	200	X	Reusable
	Lithotriptor baskets	Dormia	Monofilament	Stainless steel	4	15, 20, 25, 30, 35	200	O	Reusable
	Stone extraction baskets	Dormia	Monofilament	Stainless steel	4	20, 25, 30, 35	120, 200, 260	X	
	Stone extraction baskets	Spiral	Monofilament	Stainless steel	6	20	200	X	
	twist´n´CATCH-Stone extraction baskets	Dormia	Monofilament	Stainless steel	4	35	200	X	
	Lithotriptor baskets (single-use)	Dormia	Monofilament	Stainless steel	4	20, 25, 30, 35	200	O	
	Rock star (single-use)	Dormia	Monofilament	Stainless steel	4	35	190	O	
MTW Endoskopie	Lithotomy basket twisted wires	Dormia	Monofilament	Stainless steel	4			△ (rescue)	
	Lithotomy basket turned	Dormia	Monofilament	Stainless steel	4			△ (rescue)	
	Lithotomy basket 6 wires turned	Fogarty	Monofilament	Stainless steel	6			△ (rescue)	
	Lithotomy basket 6 wires turned	Fogarty	Monofilament	Nitinol	6			△ (rescue)	Guidewire assisted
	Lithotomy basket diamond shaped	Diamond	Monofilament	Stainless steel	4			△ (rescue)	
	Lithotomy basket for guide wire	Fogarty	Monofilament	Stainless steel	4			△ (rescue)	Guidewire assisted
Olympus	Flower Basket V rotatable type	Fogarty	Monofilament	Stainless steel	8	20	190	O	Ball tip
	Flower Basket V wire-guided type	Fogarty	Monofilament	Stainless steel	8	20	190	O	Guidewire assisted
	Tetra Catch V rotatable type	Fogarty	Monofilament	Stainless steel	4	22	190	O	Ball tip
	Tetra Catch V wire-guided type	Fogarty	Monofilament	Stainless steel	4	22	190	O	Guidewire assisted
	LithoCrush V wire-guided and rotatable type	Dormia	Monofilament	Stainless steel	4	26,30	190	O	Guidewire assisted
Taewoong Medical	Optimos Stone Basket	Dormia	Monofilament	Stainless steel	4	15, 20, 30, 40	250	O	
	Optimos Stone Basket	Fogarty	Monofilament	Stainless steel	8	20, 30	250	O	
	Optimos Stone Basket	Spiral	Monofilament	Nitinol	8	20, 30	200	X	

06 Stone extraction balloon

Balloon extraction catheter

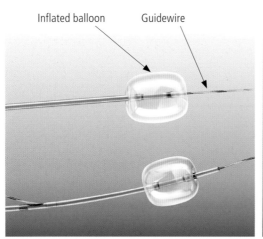

Inflated balloon   Guidewire

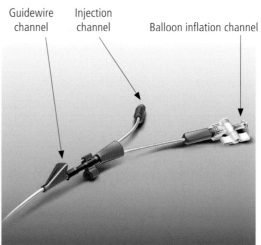

Guidewire channel   Injection channel   Balloon inflation channel

Table 6. Basic characteristics of the currently available stone extraction balloons in Korea

Manufacturer	Commercial name	Lumen number	Catheter diameter (Fr)	Catheter length (cm)	Balloon inflated diameter (mm)	Injection site (above balloon vs. below balloon)	Recommended guidewire	Special characteristics
Boston Scientific	Extractor RX Retrieval Balloon	Triple-lumen	7	200	9-12, 12-15, 15-18	Above & below	0.035	2-step inflation
	Extractor XL Retrieval Balloon	Triple-lumen	7	200	9-12, 12-15, 15-18	Above & below	0.035	2-step inflation
	Extractor DL Retrieval Balloon	Double-lumen	7	200	9-12, 12-15, 15-18	Above	0.035	2-step inflation
Cook Endoscopy	Tri-Ex Multiple Size Extraction Balloon	Triple-lumen	7-5 (tapered)	200	8.5-12-15	Above & below	0.035	3-step inflation
	Tri-Ex Extraction Balloon	Triple-lumen	7-5 (tapered)	200	8.5, 12, 15	Above & below	0.035	
	Fusion Quattro Extraction Balloon	Triple-lumen	6.6	200	8.5-10-12-15, 12-15-18-20*	Above & below	0.035	4-step inflation Wire exits extra-hole below balloon
	Fusion Extraction Balloon	Triple-lumen	7-5 (tapered)	200	8.5-12-15	Above & below	0.035	3-step inflation Wire exits extra-hole below balloon
	Escort II Extraction Balloon	Double-lumen	6.8-5 (tapered)	200	8.5, 12, 15	Above	0.035	
Medwork	Stone extraction balloons	Triple-lumen	7	200	Up to 16	Above	0.035	
	Stone extraction balloons	Double-lumen	7	200	Up to 16	Above	0.035	
	Stone extraction balloons	Double-lumen	5-7	200	Up to 16	Above	0.035	Tapered catheter diameter
MTW Endoskopie	Balloon Catheter	Triple-lumen	7, 7>5	200	16, 18	Above & below	0.035	
	Balloon Catheter	Double-lumen	5	200	12, 16	Above	0.025	
Olympus	V-System Extraction: Multi-3V	Triple-lumen	5.5-7	190	8.5-11.5-15	Above & below	0.035	3-step inflation/ Monorail & standard type
	V-System Extraction: Multi-3V Plus	Triple-lumen	5.5-7	190	15-18-20	Above & below	0.035	3-step inflation Monorail & standard type

07 Plastic stent

Plastic stent

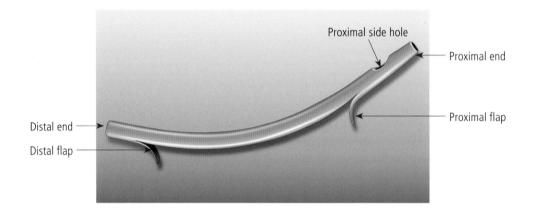

Proximal side hole

Proximal end

Proximal flap

Distal end

Distal flap

Types of biliary plastic stent

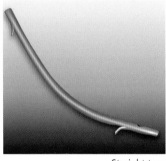
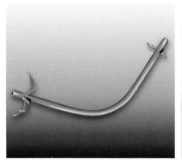
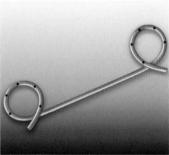

Straight type   Tannenbaum type   Double pigtail type

Types of pancreatic plastic stent

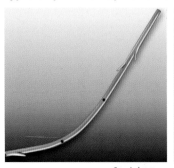
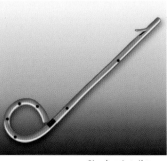

Straight type   Single pigtail type
(with or without flap)

Table 7. **Basic characteristics of the currently available plastic stents in Korea**

Manufacturer	Commercial name	Purpose	Type	Material	Size (Fr)	Length (cm)	Delivery system
Boston Scientific	Advanix™	Biliary duct	Straight type	Polyethylene	7, 8.5, 10	5-18	NaviFlex™ RX delivery system: 7, 8.5, 10 Fr
		Biliary duct	Double pigtail type	Polyethylene	7, 10	3-15	
	Advanix™	Pancreatic duct	Straight type	Polyethylene	3, 4, 5, 7, 10	2-18	RX/LW Pusher: 3 Fr, 4 & 5 Fr NaviFlex™ RX delivery system: 7, 10 Fr
		Pancreatic duct	Single pigtail type	Polyethylene	3, 4, 5, 7	2-18	
Cook Endoscopy	Cotton-Leung®	Biliary duct	Non-pigtail (flap)	Polyethylene	5, 7, 8.5, 10, 11.5	3-15	Pushing catheter: 5-11.5 Fr / Oasis® Introduction System: 8.5-11.5 Fr
	Sohendra Tannenbaum®	Biliary duct	Non-pigtail (flap)	Polytetrafluo-roethylene	8.5, 10, 11.5	5-15	
	Zimmon®	Biliary duct	Double pigtail type	Polyethylene	5, 6, 7, 10	3-15	
	Geenen®	Pancreatic duct	Non-pigtail (flap)	Polyethylene	3, 5, 7	3-15	Pushing catheter: 3~7 Fr
	Zimmon®	Pancreatic duct	Single pigtail type	Polyethylene	3, 5, 7	3-15	
	Solus®	Biliary duct	Double Pigtail	Polyurethane	10	1-15	Set Includes Introduction System (10 Fr pushing catheter, 5 Fr guiding catheter)
	Cotton-Leung® Sof-Flex®	Biliary duct	Non-pigtail (flap)	Polyurethane	7, 10	5-15	Pushing catheter: 7 Fr Fusion Oasis® Introduction System: 10 Fr

08 Metal stent

Basic structures of metal stents according to the manufacturing methods

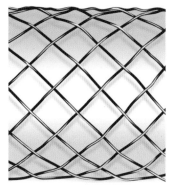

Cross wire knitting

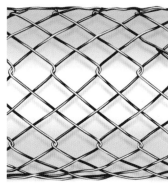

Hook and cross knitting

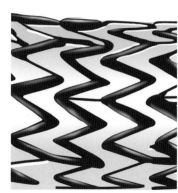

Laser cutting

Typical characteristics of metal stents

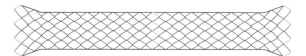

Bare metal stent

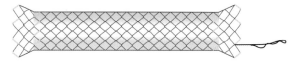

Partially covered metal stent with lasso

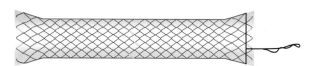

Fully covered metal stent with lasso

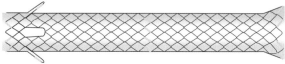

Anti-migration fully covered metal stent (single flap type)

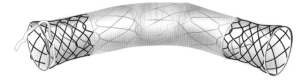

Anti-migration fully covered metal stent with lasso
(different radial forces in each segment)

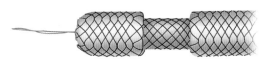

Anti-migration fully covered metal stent with lasso
(different diameters in each segment)

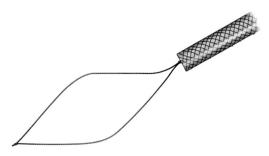

Anti-migration fully covered metal stent with long
nitinol lasso (Proximal flanged)

Bilateral stenting for hilar obstruction

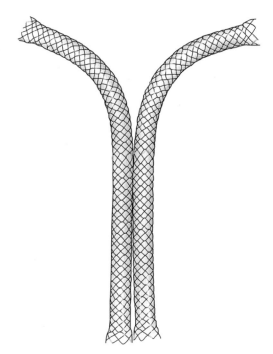

Side-by-side metal stents

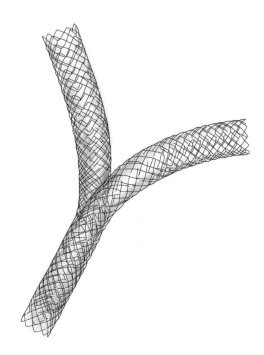

Stent-in-stent metal stents

09 Cytology brush and biopsy forceps

Cytology brush

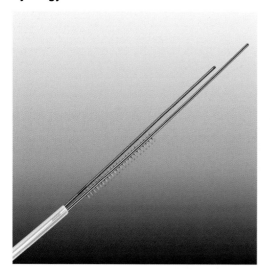

Guidewire-assisted

Biopsy forceps

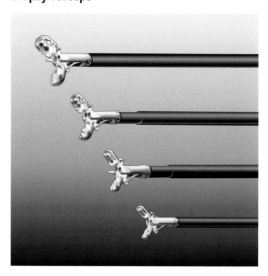

Table 9. Basic characteristics of the currently available ERCP cytology brushes and biopsy forceps in Korea

Manufacturer	Commercial name	Brush or cup diameter (mm)	Catheter O.D. (Fr)	Length (cm)	Guidewire (inch)	Special characteristics
Boston Scientific	Rx Cytology Brush	2.1	8	200	0.035	Separate guidewire lumen for exchanging accessories
	Radial Jaw 4 Pediatric Biopsy forceps	1.8	6	160/240	n/a	
Cook Endoscopy	Cytomax II® Double Lumen Cytology Brush	3.0	6 / 8	200	0.021 / 0.035	Double lumen Tip size : 1.5 / 3.5 cm
MTW Endoskopie	Cytology Brush	2.5	5.25	120		Broncho
		3.0	7.5	160		Gastro
		3.0	7.5	220		Colon
Olympus	Cytology Brush	2.4	5.6	195	0.035	
	ERCP catheter with biopsy forceps	2.0	6.5	155	n/a	Alligator jaw-step / Standard-oval

10 Naso-biliary and naso-pancreatic drainage tube

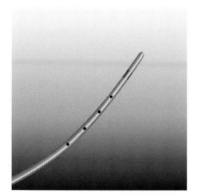

Straight type

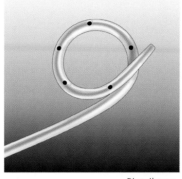

Pigtail type

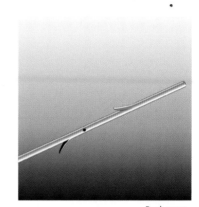

Barb type

Table 10. **Basic characteristics of the currently available naso-biliary and naso-pancreatic drainage tube in Korea**

Manufacturer	Commercial name	Purpose	Type	Material	Size (Fr)	Length (cm)
Boston Scientific	Flexima Nasobiliary Catheter	Biliary duct	Pigtail type	Polyethylene	5, 6, 7.5, 8.5	250
Cook Endoscopy	Nasal biliary drainage set	Biliary duct	Pigtail type/ Straight type	Polyethylene	5, 7	235
	Nasal pancreatic drainage set	Pancreatic duct	Barb type	Polyethylene	5	250
Taewoong Medical	Optimos™ ENBD Catheter	Biliary duct	Pigtail type/ Straight type	Polyethylene	5, 6, 7	250
	Optimos™ ENBD Catheter	Pancreatic duct	Barb type	Polyethylene	5, 6	250
MTW Endoskopie	Nasobiliary drainage catheter	Biliary duct	Pigtail type	Polyethylene	5, 7	250